Health Care as a Social Good

WITHDRAWN

Health Care as a Social Good

Religious Values and American Democracy

DAVID M. CRAIG

GEORGETOWN UNIVERSITY PRESS
Washington, DC

Library of Congress Cataloging-in-Publication Data

Craig, David Melville, 1965– author.
    Health care as a social good : religious values and American democracy / David M. Craig.
        p. ; cm.
    Includes bibliographical references and index.
    ISBN 978-1-62616-138-2 (hardcover : alk. paper)
    ISBN 978-1-62616-077-4 (pbk. : alk. paper)
    I. Title.
    [DNLM: 1. Health Care Reform—United States. 2. Public Policy—United States.
3. Religion—United States. 4. Social Justice—United States. 5. Social Values—United States.
WA 540 AA1]
RA418.3.U6
362.10973—dc23
                                                                                    2014005920

♾ This book is printed on acid-free paper meeting the requirements of the American National Standard for Permanence in Paper for Printed Library Materials.

15 14   9 8 7 6 5 4 3 2   First printing

Printed in the United States of America

To my parents,
Ann and Norman Craig

Contents

Acknowledgments

THIS PROJECT began years ago in a conversation with my cousin Curt Williams about Catholic hospitals and economic justice. Although my research expanded into many other conversations, I hope that Curt's passion for justice shines throughout the book. My interest in ethics and public policy dates back even further to family dinner conversations in my youth. My parents' engagement with public affairs and their dedication to the common good informed my desire to join the health care reform debate. Ann and Norman Craig's reflective commitment to living out their religious values is a model for the dialogue and work I foresee in the years ahead. I dedicate this book to them. My wife Jocelyn Sisson gave her constant support—intellectual, editorial, and soulful—throughout the project. Our daughters Claudia and Eliza Craig kept me going with their lively dinner banter and their cheerful inquiries into their father's mood and the book's progress.

I have more people to thank than I can name and an even longer list of people to thank whom I cannot name. This book would not be possible without my anonymous interviewees who patiently and vividly explained the complexities of health care and health policy. As a scholar, I am frustrated not to be able to credit people for their revealing anecdotes, arresting phrases, and keen insights. I extend to all of my interviewees this indirect expression of gratitude for their time, experience, and candor. I hope they hear their voice in the book, one part in a searching and morally serious civic dialogue about the present and future of health care in the United States.

My colleagues in IUPUI's Religious Studies Department encouraged me to write for a broad public. I thank Matthew Condon, Edward Curtis, Tom Davis, Johnny Flynn, Philip Goff, Kelly Hayes, Andrea Jain, Ted Mullen, Peter Thuesen, Joseph Tucker Edmonds, and Rachel Wheeler for reading chapters and offering clarifying pointers. Marc Bilodeau, Aaron Carroll, Carrie Foote, Greg Gramelspacher, Anne Royalty, Rich Steinberg, Richard Turner, and Mark Wilhelm stretched my thinking into health economics and policy, philanthropy and ethnography. Kevin Cramer sharpened my arguments with his usual discerning questions. Sarah Hamang masterfully annotated the latest health policy research, and Richard Clark connected me to local religion and healthy communities initiatives. Diana Embry and Debbie Dale expertly transcribed the interviews. I am grateful for a sabbatical leave from IUPUI, along with research support from the IU Center on Philanthropy and the IU School of Liberal Arts at IUPUI, which allowed me to conduct the interviews. I thank Bill Enright and the Lake family's generosity for the opportunity to serve as the Thomas H. Lake Scholar in Religion and Philanthropy, which enabled me to write the book.

I thank Richard Brown at Georgetown University Press for believing in and seeing my vision of the book through to the end. I appreciate the comments of the anonymous reviewers who helped focus and tighten the arguments. Chapters 4, 5, and 6 are based, respectively, on my articles "Religious Health Care as Community Benefit: Social Contract, Covenant, or Common Good?" *Kennedy Institute of Ethics Journal* 18, no. 4: 301–30; "Catholic and Jewish Ethics in the Health Care Market," *Journal of the Society of Christian Ethics* 28, no. 2: 223–43; and "Everyone at the Table? Religious Activism and Health Care Reform in Massachusetts," *Journal of Religious Ethics* 40, no. 2: 335–58. I thank the current editors of these journals and Johns Hopkins University Press, Georgetown University Press, and Blackwell Publishing for permission to reprint.

Introduction

HEARING HEALTH CARE VALUES

I'm half-kiddingly but half-seriously saying that we're going to bring the capitalists and the socialists into a room, and then we're going to have a battle royale because it's meaningless for me to go into the public policy arena saying I'm for universal coverage and that's all I can say. We're going to wake up one of these days, and health care reform in the market is going to have to happen. If you don't want that, if you don't like the entirely individualistic model, if you think it's going to leave out the poor, you should be concerned about who we are. So now is the time to engage. What are we for?

Government affairs director, West Coast Catholic health system

IMAGINE A LEGISLATURE or a town hall meeting where the "capitalists" and the "socialists" were not allowed to leave until they came to some agreement about the main goals and policies of health care reform. This scene seems impossible in the United States. The continuing debate over the 2010 Patient Protection and Affordable Care Act is less a "battle royale" than a battle without end. Despite surviving judicial review by the US Supreme Court in 2012, the law's implementation remained beset by partisan rancor. A constructive step forward would be for partisans on both sides to agree that the labels capitalist and socialist might be used in jest behind closed doors but not in public statements driven by anger, ideology, or political gamesmanship. Instead of labeling people, I propose that it is more productive and accurate to name the different ideas of health care in the national debate. Whereas many conservatives believe that health care is a private choice, many liberals believe that it is a right. Both understandings of health care can legitimately claim to serve important values, and each one is backed by a distinct vision of justice.

The health care reform debate in the United States is a debate about the kind of society that Americans want. Describing the debate in such elevated terms

1

may seem too charitable. Some liberals presume that the sole motivation behind conservative resistance to universal health coverage is crass selfishness, as if the sentiment "I have mine and you don't" is the crux of all conservative opposition to the Affordable Care Act (ACA). Similarly, some conservatives describe the push for health care reform as a power grab by "takers" whose only motivation is to enjoy a free ride at the expense of "makers." Ascribing bad motives to one's opponents is commonplace in politics, but it ignores how high the stakes are in this debate.

The stakes are high because of the extreme cost of US health care and because of the extreme vulnerability that makes it essential at times. The United States devotes a much larger percentage of its annual spending to health care than do other advanced economies, and the rate of spending increase continues to out-pace inflation. As escalating costs absorb more and more of family income and government budgets, Americans face basic questions not only about the coun-try's fiscal welfare but also about its political character. One certainty is that controlling health care costs has to become a national priority. At the same time there is a widely shared recognition that health need is not restricted to people with health insurance. As a result, compassion requires making some provision for uninsured people to have access to the vast health care resources in this country. The challenges are societywide: how to control costs and how to ensure at least decent care. Recognizing how high the stakes are may help Americans find the charity needed to push past angry words and listen to the sincere values on both sides of the political debate.

I have taken the epigraph to this introduction from a government affairs director at a Catholic health care system on the west coast. He was one of a hundred people I interviewed during a journey through US health care.[1] The journey took me across the country as I listened to health care insiders who worked for nonprofit providers with a religious affiliation and to religious activ-ists who participated in an interfaith coalition that lobbied for the 2006 Mas-sachusetts health care reform law. The common denominator among my interviewees was their participation in an organization serving religious values. Of interest to me were both the religious language that shaped their discussions about how to deliver and reform health care and also the shared commitment to seeing their discussions through whatever disagreements arose along the way.

Judaism and Christianity—the two traditions I encountered on my jour-ney—offer a range of powerful visions of responsibility, justice, and commu-nity.[2] Putting these visions into practice in a religious congregation, an interfaith coalition, or a religious health care organization can help participants identify who they are, celebrate what values they stand for, and cooperate on behalf of their commitments. The same objectives inspired the government affairs director's wish to corral his organization's leadership team long enough for them to hear each other out on the ethics and the economics of US health care. Who are we? What are we for? Given our mission and values, how should we deliver health care in a competitive marketplace?

These questions presuppose a "we," a congregation, coalition, or organization with which one associates by choice. Mutual understanding and constructive compromise are hard enough to foster in an association, let alone in public deliberation about such divisive issues as reforming US health care. The motivation for this book, however, is the recognition that all of the leading arguments in the reform debate answer to visions of responsibility, justice, and community that represent the views of large numbers of Americans. The book's premise is that listening to—and actually hearing—the values of people with whom we disagree can change the conversation and chart a path toward meaningful and lasting reform.

RELIGIOUS VALUES AND AMERICAN DEMOCRACY

This book argues that religious values are vital to this public conversation for two reasons. First, US health care is already shaped by the many religious health care nonprofits that operate and deliver care in response to their mission and values. Accounting for the practical effect of those values on public policy is the purpose of the second half of the book.[3] More important for now, I propose that religious values can open a space in public discussions where liberals and conservatives may be able to move past the static battle lines of sound-bite politics to the motivating moral and political visions that are the principal source of the passions in this debate. But will inviting more passions into the debate help? If some of the passions are generated by visions of human dignity, moral responsibility, and a good society that look to scriptural and traditional authorities not shared by every American, how can religious values advance the national debate or shape public policies binding on all Americans?

This question about the proper role of religious arguments in American democracy is a polarizing subtext to many contemporary debates. In the standard media storyline and in many Americans' assumptions, when religious arguments enter the public forum, they unequivocally support the conservative position on a wide range of issues from embryonic stem cell research to gay marriage to climate change. Simply put, religious values favor conservative politics. Admittedly, it is the case today that liberals are more likely than conservatives to be skeptical about and even hostile toward religious arguments in public. But equating religious values with conservative causes is historically myopic. In the decades leading up to the civil rights movement, left-leaning religious arguments held much greater sway in American public life.[4] Just as we need to disturb the battle lines of sound-bite politics, we should also question assumptions about how Americans' religious and secular values play out in public debates.

The divisiveness of contemporary public debates has been diagnosed as a "culture war,"[5] implying that Americans' value conflicts are so entrenched as to be foundational to their sense of being and belonging. In the culture war framework, the more that public debates cross into moral terrain, the more apparent it becomes that Americans are grouped into factions with dueling visions of the good society. To borrow a biblical motif, liberals and conservatives, progressives and traditionalists, are on divergent moral journeys to their own Promised Lands. Not only do the imagined destinations differ, but getting there requires marching in step with fellow travelers and orienting all of one's ethical judgments toward the truth of one's goal. Thus each group's moral reasoning becomes so culturally insular that it is unintelligible to outsiders. Americans may speak the same words—justice, dignity, community—but it is as if they were consulting the dictionaries of different languages, for which no translations are possible.

Acknowledging the threat of a culture war, some secular liberals argue that collective moral journeys have no place in public discussion or political deliberation.[6] On this secular liberal reading of the US Constitution, We the People agree from the outset to put aside our communal moral journeys in debating, legislating, implementing, and adjudicating the laws of the land. For secular liberals, the terms of politics should be defined by a dictionary of neutral legal terms, supplemented perhaps by scrupulous political histories of the United States. The apparent neutrality of this position is shadowed, however, by two questionable premises. Secular liberals focus on religion as the source of those troublesome moral journeys, and they disavow any desire to take the country on a moral journey toward their vision of the good.[7]

The ongoing debate over the Affordable Care Act may appear to confirm these secular liberal premises. On the one hand, liberals have long argued for universal coverage in the secular languages of individual rights and cost-benefit analysis. Liberals claim that health care is a human right essential to people's ability to participate in and contribute to their society. Their economic arguments support paying the cost of universal coverage both to offer poorer patients the benefits of regular care and to avoid the wasteful expense of delivering primary care through emergency rooms and delaying treatment for chronic diseases. On the other hand, in the debate over the ACA, the United States Conference of Catholic Bishops, evangelical Protestants, and other conservative Christians raised religious objections to potential federal funding of abortion and to federal mandates that employer-sponsored health insurance cover birth control.[8] These religious objections were so pronounced that they threatened to derail the ACA until President Obama issued an executive order tightening the ACA's restrictions on abortion funding. He later conceded that insurers, not employers, were responsible for covering birth control, a concession that offered little relief to those religious organizations objecting to the mandate that also self-insure their workers.[9]

The reasonableness of these concessions lies in the eye of the beholder. Liberals cite the constitutional principle of equal protection to argue that federal rules about mandated health insurance policies must apply the same to all Americans. If the ACA's minimal coverage standards include effective contraception, as justified by a right to privacy, then equal access to this benefit must be secured for everyone regardless of whether one's employer is a secular or a faith-based organization. From this perspective, allowing expressly religious organizations to waive the mandate to cover contraception is reasonable, but equality-in-coverage guarantees must then be enforced on insurers. For conservatives this policy compromise is a case of pragmatic moral selectivity. Liberals couch their commitments to privacy and reproductive freedom in appeals to secularity while ruling other moral arguments out of bounds because of their religious overtones. It is understandable, therefore, that conservatives question whether liberals' resistance to religion in public life is more a matter of constitutional scruples or political advantage.

Mandating coverage for birth control is politically popular but socially contentious. I raise the issue not to resolve it but to foreground the social dimensions of disagreements over the proper direction of health care reform. Health care is so expensive, complex, and vital to our lives that health policy decisions tie Americans' choices and responsibilities more closely together than in other arenas of public policy. This social sharing of health benefits, risks, and costs is reflected in the hybrid character of US health care, which liberals and conservatives both overlook. The push for solutions that rely exclusively on *either* public mandates *or* private markets ignores the longstanding public-private partnerships that built and continue to fund the country's health care infrastructure and medical research and training programs. Also obscured is the role of nonprofit organizations in delivering care. The many providers with a religious name—Jewish, Baptist, Methodist, Presbyterian, Adventist, the countless Catholic saints, and so forth—testify to the historical importance of religious communities serving their values by establishing hospitals to train caregivers, provide health care, and include the excluded.[10] Nonprofit providers with both a religious history and an active religious mission are central to this study of how religious values shape US health care and why admitting the full range of these values into the national debate can help move health care reform ahead in the years to come.

The health care reform debate provides a case study of why and how the national conversation needs to change. Americans should neither resign themselves to the hopelessness of an endless culture war nor reject religious values as the source of unreasonable sectarianism in political debates. Policing collective moral journeys out of political deliberation will not do. Instead we need to look for civic spaces in which people are engaged in values-driven conversations about how to join their efforts in pursuit of good health care while seeking constructive compromise.

Religious nonprofits actively serving their mission and values resemble communities engaged in moral dialogue. In this they are similar to the interfaith coalition I visited. As these organizations deliver care or agitate for reform, participants continually discuss and debate the practical applications and moral urgency of their values. Recognizing these conduits of religious values into US health care has two implications. First, it cautions against dismissing a religious health care nonprofit's core values—for example, Catholic reverence for life on the issue of contraceptive coverage. This public disregard may weaken the organization's motivation to serve its other values, such as caring for poor and vulnerable patients, which the public encourages through tax exemptions.[11] Second, it highlights the quasi-public status of the religious values that these organizations enact, not by proof-texting biblical passages or imposing divine fiat on others, but by deliberating about an organization's shared history and religious values as its members grope their way toward constructive compromise in implementing a common mission. Simply put, religious health care providers and religious activists are on moral journeys of a sort, but their religiously informed visions of good health care have a civic status and public accessibility that seem out of place—and out of bounds—in a secular liberal ideal of reasonable political deliberation.

Progressive health care reform seeks continued progress toward guaranteed coverage for everyone in the United States. In addition to full inclusion, progressive reform requires fairness, efficiency, and sustainability to realize the goal of affordable, quality health care for all. Yet secular arguments for universal health coverage have proven weak in motivating reform in the United States, as demonstrated yet again by the deep political ambivalence toward the ACA. In my judgment, liberals have failed to persuade the American public partly because they cede values talk—particularly about religious values—to conservatives upon entering the public sphere.

The avoidance of religious values when discussing health care is especially shortsighted. Health care touches our human vulnerability, and it heightens our interdependence in mutual aid. Religious teachings, stories, symbols, and rituals foreground vulnerability and interdependence in community as secular political principles do not. In liberal traditions of politics, rights inhere in individuals as powers. Social provision for fellow citizens requires prior consent of the governed. These democratic protections of personal liberty are essential to the system of limited government in the United States, but they also reinforce the individualizing tendencies of secular political philosophies on both the left and the right. They also distract attention from the hybrid character of US health care and the solidarity in community required for progressive health care reform.

Americans prize independence, which quickly falters when health crises hit. At these times it becomes vividly, and sometimes painfully, clear how much our life journey depends on others. The cost and complexity of health care mean that family and friends are not sufficient. The mission and values of religious providers offer evocative testimony to the need for a more encompassing collective moral journey in health care. Caring for the poor and the vulnerable, stewarding resources to build up a common good in health care, fulfilling the covenantal duties of the health professions, treating patients with the respect and justice that human dignity deserves—these phrases capture some of the ways that Catholic, Protestant, Jewish, Muslim, and other religious health care organizations have put their values into practice.[12] Religious values are made practically concrete as employees work them out in the delivery of care. They take on a civic significance as administrators and caregivers with differing political perspectives debate and implement their organizational values together. Similarly, when activists pursue their religious values in serving communities or lobbying for public policies, they give public expression to the values of a religious group. By listening in on the dialogues occurring inside religious health care organizations and among interfaith activists, I learned how US health care and health policy both serve and frustrate a wide range of values—secular and religious, moral and economic.

In this book I examine all of the leading arguments in the health care reform debate, taking seriously their visions of justice and their core values. A careful examination reveals that none of them matches how US health care has been structured. Health care has not been organized as a private benefit, a private choice, or a public right so much as a social good.[13] Simply put, the social pooling of resources and costs, the social lottery of risks and needs, and the social priorities of wellness, prevention, and access to cost-effective care reflect the ways that US health care is already a social good, however incomplete. Listening to the religious values of health care leaders and activists is a first step toward clarifying the visions of justice behind conservative and liberal approaches to reform. The next step is learning how religious health care employees and religious activists are acting on their values. Both groups have created civic spaces in which people come together to enact shared values and are sometimes transformed in the process. Readers can assess the fruits of their efforts and, I hope, invest themselves in turning the hidden ways that US health care already operates as a social good into explicit public priorities. By assessing how religious values might figure in the coming decades of health care reform, this book critically examines the ethical foundations of conservative arguments for market reform and liberal arguments for health care rights. Finding both approaches wanting, I develop a moral basis for a progressive vision of health care as a social good.

THE MORAL LANGUAGES OF US HEALTH CARE

The best way to name the competing ideas of health care in the reform debate is to start with the language of ordinary Americans. I identify three moral languages that Americans speak in talking—and thinking—about health care. I call them "moral languages" because, in naming what health care is, people make assumptions about how it should be provided, paid for, and delivered. In the United States health care is viewed as (1) a private benefit, (2) a public right, and (3) a private choice.

The everyday expression "private health benefits" remains Americans' primary moral language, and it reveals much of the moral history of health care in the United States. The private benefits idea is so familiar that Americans do not realize how curious it is. Its origins lie in the institution of employer-sponsored health insurance in the United States. Starting in the middle of the twentieth century, a growing number of employers began offering more generous health insurance benefits to their employees. The term "benefits" simply designates that employer-paid insurance premiums are in addition to employee wages. The term "private" describes the voluntary basis of these insurance policies: employers and employees contract certain benefits, and employers and insurers contract the coverage terms or, increasingly, the service provisions. Although Americans have become accustomed to the institution of private health benefits, it is unique among industrialized countries.

The private benefits idea is also an odd fit with today's US health care system. The idea that work earns benefits continues to operate as a powerful moral norm in public debates, even though only half of Americans (49 percent) were covered through an employer in 2010.[14] The hold of this norm is clearest in the misperceptions surrounding the federal Medicare program. Despite being a social insurance system, in which generations of younger workers support senior citizens' health care, Medicare is popularly viewed as a private benefits system, in which seniors are due a personal payout on a lifetime of Medicare taxes. The private benefits idea also excuses the prevalence of uninsured Americans among the poor who are assumed not to work or not to work sufficiently productive jobs. Although the moral language of private benefits remains the dominant vocabulary used by Americans talk about health care, its many inadequacies include the lack of private coverage for every American, let alone for every working American.

For many liberals the moral response to these systemic deficiencies is to institute a right to health care—our second moral language. Whether conceived as a human right or a civil right, this public right would guarantee every citizen (or person living in this country) covered access to health care services. Currently there is no public right to health care in the United States, nor does the ACA codify one. In fact, the law's proponents went out of their way to reassure covered Americans that nothing would change in their health care if they were happy with their current coverage, presumably because a universal right to health care is seen as too threatening to the private benefits idea.

This political pragmatism sits uneasily with the moral arguments behind the language of health care as a public right. In the standard arguments either the right to health care inheres in human dignity or it is intrinsic to effective liberty. For example, many American denominational statements call for a right to health care as essential to the human dignity that flows from being created in God's image. In these religious arguments every neighbor suffering from disease and disability deserves reverent respect in the form of caring for them, promoting their well-being, and supporting their participation in community. The ubiquity of liberal Christian and Jewish support for a right to health care belies the notion that religious values only support conservative causes. Secular liberal arguments, for their part, often link universal coverage to personal liberty. The government must grant every citizen a right to health care because "fair equality of opportunity" does not exist, to cite two representative arguments, without the "primary good" of health care or without the "species-typical normal functioning" that health care helps maintain.[15]

Although moral considerations lead the way in these religious and secular arguments, politics and economics have to define the scope and content of the right once established. It is this secondary phase of specifying and limiting a right to health care that has made this moral language a sideshow in the national debate. An unlimited right of covered insured access to every health care service would bankrupt the nation. Setting limits, however, requires political processes for capping health care budgets and advisory boards for steering resources toward cost-effective care. Such policy tools have been used infrequently in the United States, as in Oregon's short-lived Medicaid reforms in the 1990s and, to potentially greater effect, in Massachusetts' 2012 cost-control law. Such exceptions confirm the rule that, to date, many covered Americans fear that a universal, limited right to health care will curtail their benefits. Whereas the moral language of health care as a public right is frequently sounded as a clarion call to change, in the absence of a viable implementation plan, it quickly reduces to a slogan.

The newcomer to the national debate is the third moral language—health care as a private choice. Although personally choosing one's own doctor, care, and insurance harks back to the "good old days" of independent physicians and inexpensive catastrophic health insurance, the conservative proponents of this language imagine a reinvention of US health care. Driving the transformation would be empowered consumers and innovative providers. In this model, consumer choice means selecting the health coverage and health care services that one values for the money, all the way up to the first several thousand dollars of services of a high deductible. Provider choice means organizing and pricing health care services free from the middlemen of US health care—big insurers and government programs. In a market-driven future, innovative providers would follow the lead of choosy consumers as they rewarded better health care value for the money.

The fuller implications of the language of private choice come into focus by contrasting it with the languages of private benefits and public rights. On the one hand, private choice breaks the moral link between health benefits and gainful employment. Personal responsibility alone justifies having health care choices. On the other hand, private choice rejects bureaucratic decisions by public officials about which covered services consumers should value and how much providers should be paid. Instead, individual consumers would be free to evaluate which covered services suit their risks, determine their comfort levels with deductibles and copays, and reward innovative providers of the affordable, quality care that fits their needs.

The language of private choice is a moral language, even though its proponents prefer the economic descriptors "market-driven reform" and "consumer-directed health care." The market reformers' economic goals of price and quality transparency in health care services, efficient resource allocation in response to consumer needs, and market discipline in controlling health costs advance moral values. Consumers would have incentives to save money by taking personal responsibility for their health and making prudent health care decisions. Providers would have incentives to be more responsive to chronic disease and disability where suffering is acute, poor people are disproportionately affected, and profits may be greatest. In addition to rewarding values of thrift, prudence, and even compassion, the idea of health care as a private choice answers to a vision of a just meritocracy, in which personal choice dictates the justice of owning health coverage and purchasing health care services. Any other services that physicians or hospitals choose to offer without compensation is simply charity. If consumer discipline succeeds in driving down health care costs, then even this need for charity care will abate, too, market reformers predict.

These thumbnail sketches of the three languages of US health care shift the focus from the ideological labels that caricature the participants—"capitalists" and "socialists"—to the moral visions that clarify the stakes for the United States. Of course, political caricatures can have a ring of truth. Indeed, market reform has the appearance of unbridled capitalism without a safety net. But market reformers propose changing, not eliminating, Medicare and Medicaid. Similarly, government mandates to purchase health insurance and standardize minimal coverage further "social-ize" health care risks, costs, and benefits among more Americans. But the ACA does not increase government ownership of health plans or provider organizations, the standard definition of socialized medicine.

Lost in the ideological labeling is the government affairs director's question at the top of this chapter: Is health care more an individual responsibility or a social responsibility? Market reformers want to replace social responsibility with individual responsibility; they seek to de-socialize US health care. This goal is clearest in their proposal to offer Medicare recipients fixed levels of "premium support" (vouchers) to buy private insurance on their own. Making senior citizens into health care consumers would increase their individual choices. Capping the vouchers' annual growth would enlist seniors in cost control. Thus individual decision making would replace the social pooling of risks and costs in the Medicare program. By contrast, the ACA builds on the existing social mechanisms for sharing health risks and health care costs in the United States. For example, the individual mandate, the law's controversial requirement that Americans must obtain coverage or pay a tax penalty, directs additional funds into private insurance pools or the federal health care budget. This individual responsibility is cushioned by the ACA's subsidies for families earning up to 400 percent of the federal poverty level to help them buy coverage through state health insurance exchanges. Thus as individuals assume personal responsibility for paying into US health care, they become eligible for social subsidies funded by public coffers.

This glimpse into the competing approaches of market choices versus public mandates reinforces the question of whether health care is more of an individual or a social responsibility. Market reform shifts responsibility from the social sphere to the individual, retooling the two largest public insurance programs around individual choices and private insurance. The ACA shifts responsibility in the opposite direction, using public mandates and subsidies to establish health coverage as a social norm. Although partisans ridicule each other as ideologically bound to the singular tool of market choices or public mandates, answering the perennial question of responsibility that lies at the heart of health care requires careful examination and balancing of a range of moral and economic values. Identifying the values and the visions of justice behind the three moral languages of US health care will lead to a more productive and honest conversation.

STORIES OF HEALTH POLICY

This chapter's epigraph highlights another unexpected question. How many Americans actually oppose the goal of universal coverage? I expect that in the abstract few Americans do not want their fellow citizens to have health coverage. Opposition to universal coverage is aimed, rather, at the policy means by which this goal is to be achieved: for example, a single-payer government health plan, the individual mandate, tax hikes to fund expanded coverage, or reimbursement limits on therapies, drugs, and devices that are proven to be less cost-effective through evidence-based medicine. Whether or not their concern is justified, many Americans fear a government "takeover" of US health care, "redistributive" tax policies to pay for new "entitlements," and the "rationing" of care. Inside the health care industry, however, universal coverage is welcomed with open arms so long as someone else is footing the bill. As a Jewish health policy expert from the Greater Boston Interfaith Organization told me, access is the easy part: "Everyone is for better access."[16] The Catholic government affairs director echoed this point, adding: "It's meaningless for me to go into the public policy arena saying I'm for universal coverage and that's all I can say."

These statements should not be passed over too quickly. In the interview setting I tended to hear them and move onto the next question. Their simplicity and matter-of-fact quality make it easy to miss their surprising power to shock expectations. Indeed, for advocates of health care as a public right, the struggle is all about guaranteeing universal coverage. From their perspective, a major Catholic hospital system's public advocacy for this goal should carry political clout, and the existence of a moral consensus among Catholic provider organizations that universal coverage is essential to the common good should send a powerful message to policymakers. At the start of my interviews, I made similar assumptions about the direct translatability of religious support for health care reform. I went seeking moral arguments to bring to the national debate. Yet in being exposed to the tensions between ethics and economics inside provider organizations, I learned that moral values must always be weighed against economic values.

In the United States religious providers operate in a competitive health care marketplace, not a moral bubble. A salutary skepticism about economic incentives in health care is therefore critical. Economically, universal coverage would be a boon for providers if it meant increased funding to pay for the uncompensated care received by uninsured people and no decrease in the reimbursements for other people's care. Likewise, insurers would welcome larger cash flows through their claims department. Privately insured patients would be happy to stop subsidizing other people's care through higher premiums and inflated charges. But who would pay the tab in the absence of effective cost control? The common good is a closed circle. Greater benefits for everyone come with greater burdens to share, too. It *is* meaningless to go into the health care reform debate and declare, "I support universal coverage, and that's all I can say."

Arguments for a universal right to health care are not so simplistic. Their goals are more modest, and policies for limiting costs and promoting wellness, prevention, and cost-effective care are built into the arguments. Yet the arguments tend to be deductive, starting with religious or philosophical principles and deriving a just health care system from them. As a result, the arguments remain abstracted from the economics, policies, and other practicalities of US health care. The same criticism applies to the languages of health care as a private benefit and health care as a private choice. Most Americans' ways of speaking about health care match only part of the larger reality. But by listening to people who deal daily with the question of how to serve their mission and values in a competitive health care industry we can begin to hear more clearly both the health care reform debate as a whole and the voices of people who can offer solutions.

Instead of beginning with first principles of health care justice, this book explores US health care through stories of health policy. At the micro level I draw from the anecdotes, examples, hopes, and fears recorded in my interviews as people sought to tell the story of their organization's mission and values. At the macro level I examine the record of the public values that previous generations of elected representatives have written into the country's health policies. In both contexts people draw on and debate the stories of their religious and political traditions and their organizational and national histories in hammering out health policies that are economically viable in a competitive industry and politically feasible in American culture.

By focusing on stories of health policy, this book differs from other studies of health care reform that draw on stories of individual patients' experiences with health care.[17] Using stories of patients' struggles with health care access, cost, and quality is an immediate and revealing way to invite readers' empathy. Such studies are important because empathy is vital to the health care reform debate. The financing and delivery structures are so vast and the policy arguments are so abstract that it is difficult to build moral commitments to reform without person-to-person empathy. The problem with this approach, however, is that it tends to stop at person-to-person identification. The urgent needs of uninsured individuals command all moral concern, crowding out understanding of how the financing and delivery of health care actually work. Lost are the ethical implications of the organizational, market, and policy structures of US health care, which are the focus of this book. Keeping the focus on health policy demonstrates the extent to which US health care is already organized as a social good. A central thesis of this book is that Americans have helped build US health care together through more than a half century of public policy, yet they do not recognize the extent to which they have bought in to one another's care.

THE REALITIES OF HEALTH ECONOMICS

Health care reform involves more than religious values, moral languages, and stories of health policy. It must also address the realities of health economics. Economists prize empirical clarity, and they try to avoid normative biases in their terminology. My use of the term social good, with its links to moral values, will likely raise questions among economists. Their theory of goods revolves around a central distinction between private goods and public goods.[18] Since much of the health care reform debate turns on whether private markets or public mandates are the best way to organize care, perhaps the first question to ask is whether US health care is a private good or a public good.

Some definition of terms is in order. Economists distinguish private goods and public goods based on two empirical properties of consumption—rivalry and excludability. A good is "rival" if one person's consuming it means that no one else can. Ten minutes of a physician's time is rival, as are a hospital bed and a dose of flu vaccine. Without additional supply, only one person at a time can consume the good. In addition, a good is "excludable" if its consumption can be restricted, normally by charging a fee and excluding the people who do not pay. It is harder to find clear-cut examples of excludability in US health care. Coveted spots in medical schools and nursing schools are excludable because of limited admissions. Physician visits, outpatient procedures, diagnostic tests, pharmaceutical products, medical devices, and other services are all excludable in principle because they have a price tag. Under US law, however, emergency departments must make some uncompensated care available to people who cannot pay for services through health insurance or out-of-pocket spending.

In economic theory a private good is both rival and excludable; a public good is neither rival nor excludable. It is worth observing that this terminology places all of the negatives on the public good side. The economic premise is that if consumers value a good enough to pay for it, it will be produced for sale on the market. A typical private good, such as plastic surgery, provides enough satisfaction to motivate some consumers to buy it and makes enough profit to motivate sellers all along the production chain. By contrast, a public good like the basic science behind medical research does not "pay" because there is no easy way to exclude consumers (e.g., pharmaceutical companies) from using the published results. Furthermore, because a public good can be shared by many consumers at once without diminishing its usefulness, consumers tend to undervalue it. So with sellers unmotivated to produce public goods and with consumers undervaluing them, markets fail to supply enough of them to meet consumers' actual preferences. This is an example of what economists call "market failure." To put the point sharply, what makes something a public good in economics is failure—the failure to meet consumer demand. The usual market mechanisms for satisfying consumers' preferences fail, and either the government or nonprofit organizations must step in by default to pay for or produce the desired public goods.[19]

With the distinction between private and public goods before us, we can see that it offers limited assistance because US health care is a complex mixture of both.[20] On the public good side, public funding has supported basic medical research, medical training for physicians and nurses, hospital and clinic construction, and many public health initiatives from food safety inspections to flu vaccine production to primary care clinics in underserved areas. The goods of research knowledge, high-quality training, health care infrastructure, and public health all tend toward the nonrival end of the spectrum. Furthermore, even such rival private goods as hospital beds, physician visits, and medical technology are made effectively nonexcludable through massive public spending on Medicare, Medicaid, veterans' benefits, uncompensated care pools, and other programs. The pooled funding of private group insurance further extends the availability of expensive services to people who could never afford them on their own. Thus, although in theory much of health care is rival, in practice US health care is excludable only by degrees. The economists' private good/public good distinction teaches that health care in the United States is a tangled mixture of private and public goods, largely paid for through pools of private insurance and flows of public funding.[21]

There is another way of thinking about public goods. In democratic societies elected representatives deliberate about *the* public good and pass laws meant to serve whatever common purposes manage to gain majority support and survive constitutional review. To this way of thinking, such public goods as environmental safety, universal education, and national defense are deliberately defined and proactively produced; they are not supplied reactively in response to market failure. I approach public policy from this perspective. Democratic voting and legislative deliberation establish the "shared" values that citizens can agree upon through political dissent and majority rule within the limits of the Constitution. In viewing public policy through the lens of deliberative democracy, I read the history of health policy in the United States as a process of building and adjusting US health care around the values that Americans have legislated their health care to serve.

Nevertheless, I recognize that the economic approach has several advantages. First, it is precise in predicting, on the basis of empirical properties, which goods are more or less likely to be supplied by markets. This descriptive focus helps to specify in a relatively uncontroversial way a limited but important role for government. The mixed public good/private good structure of US health care also helps account for the ample contributions made by nonprofit hospitals and health care providers, another reason why religious providers are central to this book.

Second, the economic approach is agnostic about *the* public good, which economists insist is not their business to define. Their focus is on individuals as consumers not as citizens. Thus the economists' skeptical question is always, Do public policies produce the goods that people want in the most efficient ways? As we shall see, some health policies fall short of two standards: (1) responsiveness to the informed preferences of health care consumers and (2) efficiency in the delivery of quality care for the money.

Finally, and most importantly, the economic approach fits the market-first, policy-later predisposition of American political culture with its exceptionalist emphasis on personal liberty. I name this connection between the assumptions of economic theory and the individualism of American culture not to reject either one. Rather, I base my evaluation of the prospects for lasting health care reform on this cultural ground. The long record of attempts to achieve universal coverage through a single-payer national health plan, a structure of managed competition, or, most recently, a competitive public option reflects more than obstructionism by conservative politicians.[22] Many Americans remain skeptical of assigning policymakers and oversight boards the tasks of setting global budgets, evaluating cost-effective medicine, and allocating health care resources on that basis. As a result, comparisons to other countries' health care systems, where such policies predominate, are largely beside the point. These comparisons are absent from this book. I am persuaded that the path to reform in the United States must build on the current mixed structure of private health insurers, nonprofit, for-profit, and public providers, and public funding of Medicare, Medicaid, and subsidies for mandated individual coverage.

The Affordable Care Act takes this template and initiates an experiment in strengthening the social structures of US health care. The ACA's skeleton of public policies is insufficient to the task of reform, however. Successful policy requires political legitimacy, which flows from people's active assent. Political divides will not easily disappear, though there is reason to hope that they are not permanent, because once-divisive health policies of the past, such as Medicare, are now widely accepted. For the experiment of the ACA to succeed, Americans will have to hear out the moral and economic values that different parties bring to the national debate. Hearing how religious providers and religious activists are applying their values to health care delivery and reform opens up the conversation to the shared moral commitments and civic spaces already operating within US health care. Hearing the echoes of the legislative values written into established health policy helps preserve the national priorities already made. Examining the histories of mission-driven health care and deliberative health policy in the United States, we discover a record of social norms, public values, and a commitment to our shared humanity as Americans. This record testifies to a hidden solidarity implicit in US health care. I believe that summoning forth this solidarity is essential to steering health care reform toward the goal of affordable, quality care for all.

CHAPTER OVERVIEWS

The chapters in part one cut through the ideological acrimony of the reform debate to the underlying public philosophies of health care justice. Market reform of health care is very much alive in the United States. Chapter 1 explains why private choice has become the dominant language for conservatives. In challenging the language of private benefits from the right, market reformers argue that health care should be made completely private. This chapter develops the strong economic and justice arguments in favor of market reform—specifically, that consumer choice, personal responsibility, provider innovation, and insurance deregulation will drive down the cost of US health care and eliminate the sharing in other people's health risks and health care costs that market reformers view as inefficient and unfair. Appreciating the power of this vision of health care justice is critical to a more constructive health care reform debate.

Chapter 2 turns to liberal Christian and Jewish denominational statements, which have long advocated for a universal right to decent health care as fundamental to human dignity. The social basis of Christian and Jewish visions makes shared duties of healing a moral obligation of covenant or common good. In addition, the religious image of health as wholeness has the potential to shift priorities toward prevention and wellness in community-based care. Despite their social visions of health and healing, however, most religious denominations foreground rights language when discussing health care. The more that religious liberals stress the right to health care, the more that they come into conflict with conservative Christians' defense of the right to life, decreasing support for health care reform. Furthermore, given Americans' allergy to limiting rights through public policy, the right to decent health care for all threatens to become an unlimited right to all health care. For these reasons, I urge liberals to set aside the language of health care as a public right.

One major obstacle to the ACA's full implementation is that conservatives and liberals both approach reform in the dominant American political vocabulary of individual rights. Conservatives draw those rights narrowly as contracted private services, while liberals construe them broadly as public guarantees. This private-public dichotomy makes health care justice either a private responsibility or a public responsibility, not a shared responsibility. The resulting political struggle between market choices or government mandates as *the* policy tool of reform ignores the social character of US health care, which binds Americans together in the benefits and costs of a vast health care economy, whether they realize it or not. Chapter 3 reviews the past and present of US health policy to introduce the language of health care as a social good. The public financing of the nation's health care infrastructure, medical research and training, public insurance programs, and uncompensated care reflects the unspoken solidarity that Americans have shown in building US health care together.

Part two shifts from the visions of health care justice in the national debate to ways that religious values already structure US health care. Each chapter explores a practical question and an underlying moral tension. Chapter 4 asks, What social responsibilities do Americans have to uninsured and underinsured people who need health care? Instead of answering in the abstract, I explore the policy debate over the community benefit standard, the legal requirement that nonprofit providers must satisfy to retain their tax exemption. The participants in this debate presuppose three distinct models of how community benefits should be provided: social contract, common good, and covenant. Delineating these moral models clarifies why the critics and the defenders of religious non-profit providers frequently speak past each other. A comparison of the models recommends the Catholic model of the common good as the best method for developing policies to replace reactive charity care in hospitals with proactive care in communities.

Chapter 5 assesses the prospects for market reform, asking, How far can consumer-directed health plans and physician entrepreneurship advance the goal of affordable, quality health care? I omit the phrase "for all Americans" because market reformers rank choice over access. In their view, market choice must lead the way in bending the cost curve downward through personal investments in wellness and through the integration of care around chronic disease management. Once this transformation is complete, then access to affordable, quality care for all Americans can follow. This prediction obscures a second moral tension—namely, that health care is organized as both a market commodity and a basic good in the United States. While the profit motive drives much of the financing, delivery, and development of US health care, emergency care is legally guaranteed as a basic good, and other public and provider policies reinforce this norm. The market reforms currently under way are squeezing out the internal subsidies that have offset some of the expense of uncompensated care. As market efficiency drives out more of this backdoor funding, the social costs of caring for the uninsured will still be passed onto the public, only at higher levels. The single-minded pursuit of economy without a commitment to solidarity cannot serve even the market values of transparency, responsiveness, and efficiency.

Chapter 6 takes a final step from policy realm to marketplace to political debate. How might social justice commitments to an inclusive, fair, efficient, and sustainable health care system be made meaningful to more Americans? Successfully navigating a third moral tension between commutative justice and social justice depends on opening the public debate to religious values. Commutative justice in health care means getting back the equivalent of what one put in; social justice requires cooperating to meet legitimately shared needs and costs. Americans acknowledge the pull of social responsibility in health care. Free clinics, religious hospitals, the federal law guaranteeing emergency access all speak to the social obligations that Americans have assumed in reducing the unmet health needs of the uninsured. Efforts to institute solidarity through public policy, however, confront core American beliefs in the limits of federalism, the supremacy of personal liberty, and the efficiency of markets. These political and economic articles of faith are so powerful that moving toward a socially just American health care system will take equally evocative visions of a community responding to shared vulnerability. I argue that religious languages and community engagement are necessary to engender this solidarity, using as evidence GBIO's contributions to the Massachusetts health care reform campaign. A wider interfaith movement is needed to foster the active solidarity for national health care reform that secular liberal and economic arguments have not produced.

The conclusion offers an overview of the policy tools and goals of the Affordable Care Act, taking up the critical challenge of controlling the costs of US health care. The ACA avoids both the public allocations of a single-payer system and the free play of individual preferences in market reform. Instead, it lays the policy foundation for a novel effort at social stewardship, in which Americans work out the priorities and limits that they can live with in promoting health and wellness together. Critical questions include: What mercy is owed to Americans who meet their obligation under the individual mandate? Where do charity and justice begin and end for Americans and immigrants who remain without coverage? How can we protect human dignity and advance social solidarity while stewarding limited health care resources? Addressing these complex issues requires hearing out and acting on the range of competing values. I sketch model conversations, liturgies, actions, and partnerships that religious congregations and providers can undertake in serving their values and promoting community care.

NOTES

1. This study (0506-65B) was approved by the IUPUI/Clarian Institutional Review Board on July 28, 2005. Confidentiality agreements prevent me from naming the interviewees or the health care organizations in the study.

2. Over three years, I visited eight states across the country. Interviewees included administrators, sponsors, caregivers, and other employees of Catholic and Jewish health care organizations, along with Jewish, Catholic, and Protestant activists who belonged to or worked with the Greater Boston Interfaith Organization (GBIO). Most of my interviewees worked for Catholic hospital systems, which generally focus more resources, time, and reflection on mission and values. There are many other mission-driven religious providers that I could not include due to time constraints.

3. Dougherty observes that moral values are characterized by "ubiquity, vagueness, implicitness, spontaneity, emotional charge, practicality, and depth" (*Back to Reform*, 20–24). Religious values can be even more nebulous and powerful. Giving them concrete and shared meanings is challenging in a pluralistic society, which is why the practical dialogues about mission and values in religious health care nonprofits and interfaith activist coalitions are such an important resource for a values-informed debate about health care reform.

4. See, for example, Hauerwas, "Christian Critique of Christian America."

5. See, for example, Hunter, *Culture Wars*. Hunter does not identify conflicts between religiosity and secularity as the basis of the culture war he describes and diagnoses.

6. Not all secular liberals reject religious reasoning in public deliberation about health care justice. Gutmann and Thompson comment: "Revelation, by its nature, is not accessible to many citizens. Simply citing a revelatory source therefore has no reciprocal value, but making an accessible argument that includes citing a revelatory source is not ruled out by this criteria. . . . The source of those reasons, even if inaccessible, is irrelevant to their mutual justification" ("Just Deliberation and Health Care," 81–82).

7. For representative examples of secular liberal misgivings about the place of religious reasoning and motivations in public deliberation, see Rawls, "The Idea of Public Reason" and "The Idea of Public Reason Revisited"; Rorty, "Religion as Conversation-Stopper," and Audi and Wolterstorff, *Religion in the Public Square*. I develop a fuller response to Rawls in Craig, "Everyone at the Table."

8. Two representative statements by the US Conference of Catholic Bishops against the ACA's potential funding of abortion and its mandated coverage of artificial contraceptives are made by George "Universal Health Care" and DiNardo, "Letter on Conscience Protection." On Nov. 25, 2012, the US Supreme Court returned *Liberty University v. Geithner* to the Fourth Circuit Court of Appeals to hear arguments about whether the ACA's mandates for employer-sponsored health insurance violate religious liberty.

9. For President Obama's March 24, 2010, executive order segregating federal funds from abortion services, see www.whitehouse.gov/the-press-office/executive-order-patient-protection-and-affordable-care-acts-consistency-with-longst (accessed Nov. 13, 2012). See also Cooper and Goodstein, "Rule Shift on Birth Control Is Concession to Obama Allies."

10. For a history of Catholic hospitals in the United States, see Kauffman, *Ministry and Meaning*. For an account of the challenges of maintaining mission and values, see Arbuckle, *Healthcare Ministry*. Although mainly focused on one hospital, Newark Beth Israel, the recent volume *Covenant of Care* by Kraut and Kraut offers an insightful history of Jewish hospitals in the United States.

11. If the federal government exempted religious health care organizations from the mandate to cover free contraception, employees could still argue internally for this coverage. The federal government would set the bar with a nearly universal law, and expressly religious health care organizations that sought an exemption would have to justify themselves both to their religious sponsors and to their employees.

12. For a discussion of Muslim community-based health organizations, see Laird and Cadge, "Muslims, Medicine, and Mercy."

13. I am not the first to call health care a "social good." See, for example, Beauchamp, *Health Care Reform and the Battle for the Body Politic*, 89; Zoloth, *Health Care and the Ethics of Encounter*, 49–50; and Pellegrino, "The Commodification of Medical and Health Care," 261.

14. Kaiser Family Foundation, "Health Insurance Coverage of the Total Population." http://kff.org/other/state-indicator/total-population.

15. For discussion of the primary good of health care, see, for example, Green, "Health Care and Justice in Contract Theory Perspective"; and Green, "The Priority of Health Care." Daniels derives a right to health care from John Rawls's principle of fair equality of opportunity. He identifies species-typical normal functioning as the basis for determining which health and health care needs warrant guaranteed provision through universal coverage (*Just Health Care*, 4–9, 26–28, 78–79).

16. Although the Greater Boston Interfaith Organization agreed to be identified, I maintain the anonymity of all interviewees as a condition of this study.

17. A powerful example of using patients' stories to clarify issues in health care reform can be found in Zoloth, *Health Care and the Ethics of Encounter*, esp. 3–8. Vigen's *Women, Ethics, and Inequality in U.S. Healthcare*, a moral ethnography of African American and Latina breast cancer patients, examines the racial and ethnic disparities in health care access and health outcomes in the United States. For an examination of the narratives of patients *and* health professionals—physicians, nurses, chaplains, hospice caregivers, but not hospital administrators—see Smith, *Caring Well*.

18. Musgrave, *The Economics of U.S. Health Care Policy*, 24–25.

19. Economists would object that I read too much into the term "failure." In addition, Steinberg notes that nonprofit organizations and governments provide collective goods for reasons other than the inefficiencies of market failure. Redistributing resources for greater equity, developing people's preferences for social values, and expressing personal value commitments all apply in the case of US health care. See Steinberg, "Economic Theories," 128–29.

20. Economists have developed more fine-grained analytical concepts for addressing the mixing of private goods and public goods in US health care—e.g., "excluded collective goods" (Steinberg, "Economic Theories," 123).

21. Arrow initiated the lengthy economic literature on the role of "nonmarket social institutions" in addressing the uncertainties of risk and the asymmetries of information in health care ("Uncertainty and the Welfare Economics of Medical Care," 947).

22. For a defense of a single-payer health plan, see Beauchamp, *Health Care Reform and the Battle for the Body Politic*. Woolhandler and Himmelstein have also written extensively on the single-payer system, including Woolhandler, Campbell, and Himmelstein, "Health Care Administration Costs in the U.S. and Canada." For an overview of managed competition, see McDonough, *Can a Health Care Market Be Moral?*

Part One

The Moral Languages of US Health Care

Chapter 1

Health Care as a Private Benefit or Private Choice

Consumer-driven health care is similar to managed care back in the nineties. You may not have liked managed care, but if you weren't in it, you weren't in health care. Consumer-driven health care may be the grammar that structures the conversation in the future.

Director of mission and values, nationwide Catholic hospital system

AMERICANS ARE divided and confused about health care reform. The divisions were on display during the congressional debates and votes over the legislation that became the Patient Protection and Affordable Care Act of 2010. Alone among his fellow Republicans, Anh Cao, a Louisiana representative, voted for the original House bill. He cast the only Republican vote in favor of any of the bills that fed into the federal law. After the Senate voted along straight party lines, Mr. Cao then joined all of his fellow House Republicans and thirty-four House Democrats in voting against the Senate bill that President Barack Obama ultimately signed into law. This partisan divide and the acrimony of the congressional debate raise the question: Can Americans talk to each other about health care, let alone deliberate about how to reform it?

This question must be answered affirmatively, and there is reason for hope because the story of health care reform in the United States has finally changed. The most significant change is not the 2010 passage of the Affordable Care Act or the US Supreme Court's 2012 ruling in its favor. The decisive change is that liberals and conservatives now both recognize the need for some kind of systemic reform. With US health spending projections predicting a near doubling from $2.2 trillion in 2008 to $4.3 trillion in 2020, the question is no longer whether to reform health care.[1] It is how to reform health care in the face of unsustainable cost inflation.

Although Republicans and Democrats have both recognized this reality, they remain bitterly divided over whether market forces or government mandates should be the principal tool of reform. The policy debates over the right balance between private enterprise and government regulation employ frightening sound bites about a government takeover of health care and the greed of big insurers. Politicians are adept at crafting language that mobilizes their constituencies' anger and fear. They wave frantically at the tips of icebergs threatening the ship of state, ignoring or minimizing the real dangers that they know are lurking below the surface of the water.

Their rhetorical strategies are effective because they build on Americans' ways of talking about health care. On the one hand, some Americans hold fast to the ideal of the 1970s television character, Marcus Welby, M.D., the private family physician who is trusted with their personal health care. This iconic figure has been swept up into large group practices and specialty clinics. The result is a US health care system rife with corporate bureaucracies, but conservatives nonetheless zero in on government bureaucrats intruding on the physician-patient relationship as the quintessential threat to people's health care and personal choice. On the other hand, although Americans tend to look kindly on the private sector for providing many services, there are limits to that tolerance. The large executive salaries and corporate profits in the health insurance industry are an easily quantifiable indicator of the largesse in US health care spending. Because insurance companies provide no care, they lack the physician's defense of caring about their patients. Physicians put people first, while insurers put profits first, liberals argue, adding that only the government can tame the power of the insurance industry and protect the rights of patients too often denied the services they need.

Although simplistic, these images of unaccountable civil servants and venal insurance executives are remarkably effective. Their power lodges in their ability to tap into the root ideas of the health care languages that Americans speak. The old politics of health care reform could be mapped along a single linguistic divide with conservatives defending *private benefits* and progressives arguing for *public rights* to health care. More recently, conservatives have shifted to arguing that health care should be driven by *private choices*. The moral languages of private benefits, public rights, and private choice all carry with them assumptions about how health care should be provided, paid for, and delivered. How Americans talk about health care reflects their vision of how health care should be distributed.

This chapter begins an exploration of the moral languages of US health care. I call them moral languages because they each come with a vision of justice, community, and responsibility. Participants in the health care reform debate frequently dismiss their opponents for acting in bad faith and putting their self-interested concerns with money and power first. For example, Republicans are seen as willing to sacrifice the poor on the altar of free enterprise so that their corporate benefactors can make even more money from health care. Democrats are seen as willing to sacrifice medical innovation, personal freedom, and even human life in the interests of big government and their own political power. Such objections are too easy. They neither advance the debate nor contribute to the constructive compromises required to address both the crushing cost of US health care and the reality that one in six Americans lacked health insurance prior to the ACA's complete rollout in 2014. It is time to take seriously each side's moral language, assumptions, and arguments. I am not naively hoping that if partisans impute good faith to their opponents the divisions in Americans' views of health care reform will disappear. Fundamental convictions about the country's fiscal welfare and political character are at stake. We can, however, lessen the confusion surrounding health care reform by taking stock of the moral commitments embedded in each of the three ways that Americans talk and think about US health care.

DISTRIBUTIVE JUSTICE: FREE EXCHANGE, DESERT, AND NEED

Understanding how the moral languages of US health care relate to distinct visions of justice, community, and responsibility requires the concept of distributive justice. Distributive justice presupposes that there are goods we jointly produce, pay for, and use as a society, such as public education, citizenship, and national security. Distributive justice asks how the burdens of creating these shared goods and the benefits of enjoying them are distributed among people. Not surprisingly, there are sharp disagreements about distributive justice in American political debates. The idea is too large by itself to build much mutual understanding. We can get a better handle on its complexities by moving from the general idea to the actual principles by which people gain access to and possess shared goods.

Political philosopher Michael Walzer helpfully distinguishes three key principles: free exchange, desert, and need.[2] *Free exchange* is the principle of the perfect market. In this market all individuals enter with adequate purchasing power and complete information about the goods that interest them. Buyers choose from the many competitive goods available and pay the sellers their asking price. All that matters is the parties' freedom to accept or reject the deal and their fully informed agreement that they have struck a bargain of equal value to them.

Desert is the principle of recognized worth. This worth may be in the elevated form of distinctive honors awarded to an individual for special merit, or it may be in the general form of a basic dignity that commands equal respect for everyone. Desert is more than impartial, equal treatment of citizens under the law. It is appropriate regard that actively acknowledges a person and his or her inherent value or worthy qualities.

Finally, *need* is the principle of unmet necessities. Unlike the first two principles, which get specified through social interaction—either two parties agree on the equal value of the goods they are exchanging or one person's worth is recognized by other people—need can seem like an isolated, individual affair. Yet individuals cannot define what counts as need across their society. Necessity becomes need when it is unmet. The failure to provide may be one's own fault, others' fault, or no one's fault, but the judgment that a need is unmet looks to the standards of some group. Such judgments usually grow more contentious the larger the group becomes.

Separating the principles of free exchange, desert, and need at the outset will help sort out the practical and moral judgments implicit in how people talk about US health care. By listening to the meanings that Americans assign to health care and by examining the interplay of distributive principles in their visions of health care justice, we can penetrate the swirling political passions and the eye-glazing policy abstractions that cloud the public debate and make it hard for either side to see the good reasons behind their opponents' positions. A search for productive common ground requires a back-and-forth movement between the everyday political stances and economic concerns that people bring to the health care reform debate and the deeper convictions about justice that frequently turn it into little more than a shouting match.

To lower the heat and shed some light, this chapter and the next clarify the languages of private benefit, private choice, and public right as descriptions of US health care and evaluate their normative statements about justice. This chapter begins with health care as a private benefit and the unique history of employer-based health insurance in the United States. I then discuss how market-driven health care reform shifts the focus from private benefits to private choices.

HEALTH CARE AS A PRIVATE BENEFIT:
HISTORY AND CHANGE

The first language of US health care is health care as a private benefit. It is a sign of changing times, therefore, to hear the mission director of one of the largest hospital systems in the country say that consumer-directed health care, with its language of private choice, may be the "grammar that structures the conversation in the future." That future is not yet, however, as the loudest voices in the recent national debate spoke in the language of private benefits.

Consider these memorable words which crystalized the boiling opposition to Democrats' initial reform proposals during the summer of 2009. At one of many town hall meetings, a South Carolina retiree stood up and warned, "Keep your government hands off my Medicare."[3] Two different lessons can be drawn from these words, one negative and one positive. On the negative side, many Americans appear not to understand how extensive the government's role is in paying for health care. In 2010, public payers covered 45 percent of US health care costs,[4] with projected funding rising to 49 percent by 2020.[5] In the case of this retiree, the failure to recognize how dependent US health care is on public funding might be explained as willful blindness, the result of an ideological bias that distinguishes the deserving elderly who presumably have paid for their public insurance from the undeserving poor who do not.[6] On the positive side, Americans have firm convictions that health insurance and health care should be provided as private benefits. These convictions are entrenched in the history of US medical practice and a political culture of personal liberty and responsibility. To appreciate the vision of justice behind the private benefits idea, we must focus on the positive lesson, though clearly the primary pride in having earned one's health benefits is related to the secondary aversion to public entitlements.

Emphasizing the positive in the private benefits idea clarifies two objections to the Affordable Care Act, one from each side of the political spectrum. For Democrats the law's excise tax on so-called "Cadillac" insurance plans—plans with annual premiums over $10,200 for an individual or $27,500 for a family—unfairly changes the rules on the benefits that unions have won through collective bargaining and wage concessions. Union members are now out lost wages and face a 40 percent surcharge on premiums that exceed the law's limits, despite the benefits having been contractually earned. One of Republicans' many objections to the law is that it does not resolve the projected budget shortfalls in Medicare and Medicaid. To help cut future Medicare costs, Rep. Paul Ryan (R-WI) has proposed shifting Medicare toward a private insurance system subsidized by premium support.[7] Despite its many critics, this policy proposal is a reasonable response if US health care is indeed a private benefit. Pegging the premium support to the Medicare taxes an individual has paid would fit the logic of private benefits even better, but an average cap on government payments calculated on the basis of recipients' average contributions is a workable equivalent.[8]

These two objections to the Affordable Care Act illustrate what health care as a private benefit means in terms of distributive justice: *People deserve their contracted health benefits.* Specifically, people deserve the health coverage for which they have either voluntarily contracted with an employer or insurer or politically contracted with the government by paying their Medicare taxes. Both the emphasis on contracts and the type of contracts are essential, as we shall see.

The staying power of the private benefits idea reflects its history. Two policies from the 1940s and 1950s cleared the ground for the idea of health care as a private benefit to take hold and gain moral legitimacy. The first policy was an outgrowth of the federal government's wage and price controls following World War II. The development of private health benefits received a big boost from a policy exception that allowed companies to add and increase health insurance benefits for their workers even as wages were capped.[9] This distinction between wages and benefits remains a fixture of Americans' thinking today. Ask people what their earnings are, and they will likely state the gross income on their payroll stub. Employees pay close attention to this figure, but the total cost of health benefits rarely enters most workers' understanding, unless they are self-employed people who buy their own coverage or union workers who engage in collective-bargaining sessions. The premium, copay, and other coinsurance costs that American workers have increasingly had to shoulder do factor into people's income calculations as losses, but the premiums paid by employers remain out of view.[10] They are a "benefit," perceived as a bonus, almost a gift, from employers to employees.

This overview of the first language of US health care already presupposes several distributive principles. The contractual basis of health benefits points to the importance of free exchange in purchasing health insurance. Although not seen as wages, health benefits are part of the job contract that employees freely enter, which is why these benefits are considered to be private. But health benefits are not contracted in some morally neutral sense. They are felt to be deserved, a matter not simply of protected property rights but of personal recognition for worthy service rendered, as the affronted anger in the retiree's warning about his Medicare amply demonstrates. Curiously, the lack of attention that many employees pay to the costs of their health benefits and even the term "benefit" itself suggest a third distributive principle, that of need. Employers have a stake in meeting employees' needs for health care so the employees will remain productive, missing less work due to illness or injury. What counts as unmet necessity here is determined in each specific work environment, though also in the broader culture to the extent that employer-sponsored health insurance becomes a societal expectation with a set of customary benefits. The need principle may also account for the unspoken, but de facto gratitude that covered employees still show in not concerning themselves unduly with the large and growing bite that health insurance premiums are taking out of American paychecks. This sense of quiet gratitude may be changing, however.

Language matters morally. The term "benefit" is not some neutral legal term specifying the nonwage portion of someone's compensation; rather it suggests the proper contours of the relationship between employers and employees. Conservative market reformers have been quick to recognize and challenge the moral overtones of the private benefits language. To their credit, they have tried to break Americans of the habit of treating health insurance premiums as separate from their earnings. As Regina Herzlinger observes, "Employer-insured consumers are not motivated to shop carefully because they do not recognize that their health-insurance benefits are subtracted from their wages."[11] To teach Americans to be better managers of their health care dollars, market reformers want employees to purchase their insurance plans directly and pay much of the initial cost of their health care out of pocket. Thus instead of employers sending premiums to insurers, they would pay the health-benefit portion of wages directly to employees, allowing them to make private choices on their own.[12]

These consumer-directed health plans have high deductibles and lower premiums. They come with tax-free savings accounts into which employees and employers can make deposits for medical expenses. They are designed to give economic incentives to consumers to lower the cost of their health insurance and health care. As premiums drop, employees can retain more of their compensation. As deductibles rise, consumers have reasons to spend the first few thousand dollars (or more) of their annual health care expenses carefully, possibly reducing their health care spending and further increasing their net income. Regardless of whether this particular market-based reform would perform as predicted, it accurately identifies one of the most important prerequisites for reasonable dialogue about the future of the US health care system: Americans must become more conscious of the cost of their health insurance and health care services.

To date, Americans have shown limited but growing interest in high-deductible health plans. Although Michael Tanner of the libertarian Cato Institute boasted that in 2009 "more than 46 million Americans had consumer-directed health plans," of those, 30 million had flexible spending accounts that do not require a high deductible and should not be considered consumer-directed health plans.[13] In 2009, only 8 percent of covered workers had actual high-deductible health plans tied to a health savings account or health reimbursement account, but the figure jumped to 19 percent in 2012.[14] This growing but still limited interest speaks to the hold of the private benefits idea and the sense of security that comprehensive employer-based policies give to many Americans.

Returning to the history of health benefits in the United States, a second federal policy cemented the private benefits idea. In 1954, Congress codified the tax exclusion for employer-sponsored health insurance. This exclusion allows employers to deduct from their tax liability the full cost of the health insurance premiums they pay for their employees. In health economist Melissa Thomasson's words, the resulting "tax subsidy encouraged the growth of group health insurance, and sealed the institution of insurance in the U.S. as an employment based system."[15] The United States is alone among industrialized countries in tying health insurance so strongly to employment. Employers in other countries may funnel taxes or premiums for health insurance, but they do not preselect or self-insure the policies available to their employees.[16] The US practice of employer-sponsored insurance reinforces the cultural belief that health benefits are deserved, a just reward for sufficiently productive employment. If the cultural expectation is that contracted health benefits are one's moral due for worthy work, then lacking health insurance may be read as a sign that one's economic contributions do not merit this moral regard. Mostly, however, the private benefits idea highlights the positive rewards of having insurance while ignoring the consequences of not having it. Americans with health insurance enjoy the financial security of being insured, and they take pride in the worth of their work and in a perceived moral fairness of their health benefits.

This perception of pride and fairness is unsettled, however, by two inconvenient facts. First, most uninsured people in the United States live in families with one or more full-time workers (62 percent). Over three-quarters live in families with at least one part-time worker. Only 22 percent of the uninsured come from families where no one works.[17] The fact that work does not guarantee health benefits does not necessarily make the private benefits idea unjust because distributive justice looks at both benefits and burdens. If some types of work are insufficiently valued to command adequate compensation, then low-wage workers, it might be argued, do not contribute enough economically (a burden) to warrant expensive health insurance (a benefit). Furthermore, the push for a job with benefits drives people to invest in themselves and climb the American class ladder. Once they reach a certain rung, this line of reasoning goes, they will receive their just reward of health benefits. Yet with only 60 percent of employers offering their employees a health plan, many workers are left hanging onto the lower rungs of the ladder unable to reach the promise of private benefits.[18]

The second inconvenient fact is even harder to explain away in the name of a meritocratic conception of distributive justice. The 1954 tax exclusion for health insurance premiums applied to employer-sponsored insurance but not to the insurance policies that self-employed individuals purchase. Self-employed Americans can now deduct any medical expenses, including insurance premiums, that exceed 7.5 percent of their income. More generous is the self-employed health insurance deduction that was phased in starting in 1986, reaching a 100 percent deduction in 2003. But this deduction does not apply to Social Security taxes and some state and local taxes, leaving the self-employed relatively disadvantaged and calling into question the fairness of the private benefits idea on even a meritocratic standard of justice.[19] If equally productive (read: equally remunerative) work deserves equal treatment, then self-employed people's insurance premiums should merit the exact same tax exclusion as employer-sponsored insurance.

As the first language of US health care, the private benefit idea is backed by a powerful conception of justice, namely, that people deserve their contracted benefits because they worked for them or paid taxes to earn them for retirement. This moral principle is the backbone of the country's unique employer-based health insurance system. It also justifies the Medicare program in many people's minds, distinguishing the deserved "benefits" of Medicare from the undeserved "entitlements" of Medicaid. There are inconsistencies, however, in the justice argument undergirding the private benefits idea. Three-quarters of the uninsured live in working families, so work does not guarantee benefits. Even equally valued work does not guarantee equal treatment, as self-employed people who buy their own insurance (at higher premiums in the riskier individual markets) are disadvantaged by the US tax code. The preferential treatment of employer-sponsored insurance introduces a third inconsistency, the most challenging of all to the vision of justice at work in the language of private benefits.

Returning to the first half of Thomasson's observation about the 1954 employer-sponsored insurance tax exclusion, this policy, in her words, "encouraged the growth of group health insurance."[20] Group health insurance is a social mechanism for pooling the health risks and health care costs of a group of people. It is a social mechanism for sharing in other people's risks and costs even if the insurance is underwritten by a private company. Moreover, as health economist Uwe Reinhardt observes, most large firms base employee premiums on the average risks and costs of their workers, not on each one's health risks and cost history. He continues, "Because the arrangement forces a redistribution of income from relatively healthy to relatively sick employees, one may view [these group health policies] as miniature socialized health insurance systems."[21]

How can an employer-based system of private health insurance be socialized in any way? Although the vision of justice behind the private benefits idea is that individuals deserve the health benefits they pay for, in any given year most covered Americans contribute far more for their health insurance than they or their family use in health care. The federal government helped facilitate this redistributive social arrangement through its tax and wage policies of the 1940s and 1950s, enabling the social sharing of health risks and health care costs through employer-sponsored insurance accomplished by private companies firmly rooted in market capitalism. As history has proven, contrary to many Americans' expectations that "the private" and "the social" are antithetical, there is nothing inherently at odds between employer-sponsored private benefits and social mechanisms for insuring and funding health care.

Something similar, but less surprising, can be said about the passage of Medicare in 1965. Medicare also involves the social sharing of health risks and health care costs, in this case across the generations. A common misconception is that Medicare benefits are a return payment on a lifetime of taxes paid by recipients. In other words, senior citizens have paid for their Medicare, so the government had better keep its greedy hands off. The reality is that today's seniors receive Medicare benefits far in excess of their Medicare taxes. Calculations by Eugene Steuerle and Stephanie Rennane project that a sixty-five-year-old couple with a combined income of $86,200 in 2010 will receive a whopping 315 percent return on the "lifetime value" of their Medicare taxes, a four-to-one payout ("lifetime value" adjusts for inflation or the payout would be even higher). A forty-five-year-old couple with the same combined income in 2010 can expect less (even before any cuts to Medicare), but will still receive a substantial, if lower, return of 217 percent.[22]

Not only are Medicare benefits not fully paid for by recipients, but the distinction between deserved Medicare benefits for retirees and undeserved Medicaid entitlements for the poor rests on another misconception about who is covered by each program. Medicare covers senior citizens, people with disabilities, and people with end-stage renal disease (kidney patients needing dialysis or transplants). Medicaid covers children and adults who become eligible due to low income, which historically has been determined by the state in which they reside. Surprisingly, two-thirds of Medicaid spending in 2007 went to people with disabilities (42 percent) and senior citizens (25 percent). Thus the notion that taxpayers are bleeding to pay the health care costs of lazy working-age adults is belied by the fact that only 12 percent of Medicaid spending covers nonelderly, nondisabled adults.[23] When taxpayers share in other people's health risks and health care costs through Medicaid, they are mainly supporting the elderly and the disabled, two groups assumed to be covered by the morally acceptable Medicare program. Imagine politicians denouncing the elderly recipients of Medicaid as deadbeat freeloaders without calling down the wrath of tens of millions of senior voters. Political expedience requires the pretense that these programs serve completely different populations.

The contrasting political popularity of Medicare and Medicaid reflects both the persistence of the private benefits idea as the first language of US health care and the confusion surrounding it. Each element of the term private benefit causes confusion. On the one hand, the concept of employer-supplied benefits distracts working Americans from the fact that rising insurance premiums directly reduce their take-home pay. Getting a handle on health care inflation is in all Americans' interest, with the possible exception of those who work in the health care industry. On the other hand, the notion that health benefits are private implies that each contracted benefits package is individually owned. Most insurance coverage in the United States remains group insurance. As a result, the more that policyholders act on their perceived ownership of health care services, the less money there is available to cover their fellow policyholders' health care needs. This sense of entitlement to personal ownership of one's health benefits is widespread and growing. Nothing captures it better than the slogan "Keep your government hands off my Medicare." No doubt this attitude of entitlement is partly the product of the remarkable success of twentieth-century health policies in making comprehensive health insurance and effective medical services widely available to hundreds of millions of Americans, but this attitude is also at odds with the tacit social solidarity that built this reality. Paradoxically, the twentieth-century growth of employer-sponsored group health insurance and the popularity of Medicare indicate that most Americans embrace a social sharing of health risks and health care costs in practice, if not in name.

HEALTH CARE AS A PRIVATE CHOICE: INDIVIDUAL OWNERSHIP

Stage right: Enter the market reformers. Comparing the health care reform debate of the 1990s with today's debate, there are two notable differences on the political right. First, most opponents of the Clinton administration's reform proposals were champions of the status quo. The fretful worries of the anti-reform Harry and Louise advertisements mirrored the political strategy of

reminding Americans of the private benefits they might lose. Second, the individual mandate was originally a Republican idea. One of the proposed Republican alternatives to the Clinton bill, Sen. John Chafee's (R-RI) Health Equity
and Access Reform Today (HEART) Act of 1993, which was cosponsored by
nineteen Republican senators, included an individual mandate as a future remedy if health care access did not improve for enough Americans.[24] Now that
market reformers have become the leading conservative voices on health care
reform, they reject both the status quo and the individual mandate. For market
reformers, the status quo of private benefits must give way to the future of
private choice. Any mandate that interferes with individuals' health insurance
choices must therefore be opposed.

Market reformers recognize the paradox of the private benefits idea as practiced today. Fundamentally, market reformers reject, or at least seek to minimize, the social sharing of health risks and health care costs that structures US
health care. Earlier I mentioned Herzlinger's objection to the notion of health
insurance as a benefit. Curing Americans of their blindness to the income effects
of insurance premiums is only the start of the market reformers' agenda of
cultural change. By making us conscious consumers of health care and health
insurance, these reformers seek to replace the inconsistent justice of health care
as a private benefit with a thoroughgoing implementation of private choice in a
free market.

Market reformers have admirable consistency of conviction. When they
embrace the principle of free exchange, they mean free exchange and free
exchange alone. The contracts for health insurance and health care that they
have in mind are solely individual contracts, not the group contracts of
employer-sponsored insurance or Medicare. This subtle distinction between
individual contracts and group contracts has profound implications economically and morally, leading to a novel policy approach backed by a clear, one-
note conception of health care justice: *People own the health care services and
coverage for which they individually contract with providers and insurers.* In contrast to private benefits, the focus here is ownership largely stripped of the moral
overtones of desert that imply that health benefits are one's due. The echoes of
gift and gratitude in the provision made for workers' health care needs are also
absent from the market reformers' vision of justice.

Why, market reformers ask, does calling a good a necessity require special
provision outside of free exchange? Why, for example, should health care be
treated differently than other essential goods such as food or housing? With
food, neither employers nor the government tell people what types of groceries

they can purchase at the store.[25] Neither insurance companies nor the government dictate the prices that grocers can charge. In health care, by contrast, insurance beneficiaries must select from a short menu of policy options if they have any choice at all. Physicians and hospitals must accept the reimbursements contracted with big insurers or mandated by government programs.[26] According to market reformers, in US health care "third parties"—employers, insurers, and the government—always intrude on the market relationship between patients and caregivers, interfering with consumers' preferences and providers' prices to negative effect.[27] Freedom of choice in pricing and buying houses applies to the real estate market too, though the high cost of homeownership and the unpredictable risks of catastrophe make housing a better analogy to health care than food is. Nevertheless, profound differences remain. Homeowner policies are not comprehensive; for example, homeowners are not insured against routine maintenance of their homes.[28] Homeowners are also trusted to decide for themselves what level and what types of protection they need, and they purchase coverage out of their income, not from funds set aside by employers or the federal government.

Where food and housing are concerned, then, Americans allow direct markets between buyers and sellers to supply and price essential goods. Market reformers argue that following suit with health care would have two salutary effects. They claim that health care costs would be disciplined and that high-value care would be rewarded. The predicted effects would usher in greater efficiency in health care and consistent application of a meritocratic conception of justice.

Market reformers advocate radical changes to US health policy, including eliminating the tax exclusion for employer-sponsored insurance.[29] There are sound justice arguments and economic arguments to consider here. Starting with justice, I previously noted the unfair tax advantages for employer-sponsored insurance over self-employed insurance. In addition, both of these tax deductions are regressive: Wealthy Americans in the top tax brackets receive larger proportionate tax breaks on the health insurance premiums paid out of their compensation package or out of their personal earnings if they are self-insured. At 2012 federal tax rates, the highest income earners effectively paid only 65 percent of their health premiums (even less with state and local tax breaks factored in) because the federal government forgave 35 percent in taxes on that portion of their income. The tax break declines as workers' income drops—33 percent, 28 percent, 25 percent, 15 percent, 10 percent. So the lowest wage earners with employer-paid premiums effectively covered 90 percent, or sometimes 100 percent, of the bill out of their total compensation package. Of course, uninsured Americans received no tax break at all.

Where is the justice in giving larger tax advantages to people who earn higher incomes? Liberals who reject all market reforms, while wanting to preserve the current employer-based insurance system intact, should acknowledge the force of this justice argument. Conservatives, on the other hand, need to recognize that tax-sheltered health savings accounts and health reimbursement accounts are also regressive.[30] Furthermore, they should acknowledge that the ACA helps alleviate this injustice by creating a sliding scale of subsidies for low- to moderate-income Americans who purchase health coverage through state insurance exchanges and need help with premiums, copays, and deductibles. In effect, the new subsidies are equivalent to the tax breaks that wealthier Americans already receive. They are not handouts; they are long overdue recompense for fifty-plus years of unfairness in US tax policy.

Economists treat tax breaks and direct subsidies as one and the same. Any tax break that offsets the purchase of health insurance is effectively a public subsidy to the beneficiary, and the tax subsidies for purchasing health insurance are considerable. The nonpartisan Joint Committee on Taxation estimated that the foregone federal tax revenue from the employer-sponsored insurance exclusion was $226 billion in 2008.[31] Not only are there consequences for the federal debt, but economists argue that these subsidies distort consumers' choices about how much health insurance to purchase. If the highest income earners pay only sixty-five cents of every dollar of extra coverage because the federal government subsidizes the other thirty-five cents, then they are much likelier to accept coverage for ever more comprehensive health services despite their low value or unlikely use. The same holds true for covered taxpayers at lower tax brackets, even as their subsidy level declines. Thus the normal economic disincentives for adding marginally beneficial coverage are reduced by US tax policy, and the lost market discipline is seen as a major factor in escalating US health care costs.[32]

Market reformers share this concern about market discipline, but they emphasize another reason for weaning Americans off employer-sponsored insurance: consumer empowerment.[33] For Herzlinger, if the language of benefits gives employers too much credit for funneling employee compensation toward health insurance, then relying on employers to preselect a handful of insurance packages gives them paternalistic power in choosing covered services. Herzlinger cites the societal shift from company pension plans to employee-directed 401(k) plans as evidence that consumers can make consequential decisions about their financial security all by themselves. With adequate tools for evaluating the fees and track records of countless mutual funds, American workers have revolutionized the investment business.[34]

Market reformers seek a similar opening up of the health insurance market through two more policy changes: deregulating state insurance laws and permitting interstate sales of health insurance.[35] In this new market, consumers would no longer have to choose from a few preselected packages but could evaluate a long list of insurance options, ranging from fully comprehensive to merely catastrophic policies, unrestricted by the current barriers of state regulation. The likely effect of this change is that Americans' current group health policies and social sharing in other people's health risks and health care costs would give way to individual health policies dictated by consumers' sense of their own health risks and needs. As an example, large firms normally offer group policies that cover the prenatal services and delivery costs of a pregnancy. A portion of every worker's premiums covers services that some will never use themselves. Only rarely do firms that cover pregnancy services offer a cheaper policy without these services because doing so would prohibitively increase the cost of policies with pregnancy coverage. That is, if the pool of employees needing pregnancy care was small, the total costs of pregnancy services would be spread out across many fewer policyholders, raising the policy premiums. By contrast, an interstate market between insurers and consumers could include comprehensive policies that cover pregnancy services and a variety of leaner ones that do not. Consumers could choose the policies that covered the services they felt they needed. Why, market reformers ask, should women beyond their childbearing years and single men be forced to subsidize the costs of pregnancy for their coworkers? To take a more controversial example, fifteen states have laws requiring coverage of some infertility treatments. Why should the vast majority of state residents with no need for these services have to share in the risks and costs of expensive fertility treatments for the 7 percent of married couples who struggle with infertility?[36] Where, market reformers ask, is the justice in this distribution of burdens and benefits? Far better, these reformers argue, is to allow individuals to purchase their own health insurance, lessening the power of employers and governments and turning US health care more toward private choice.

Such objections to third-party paternalism and public mandates are justice arguments, but market reformers have economic reasons for moving toward consumer-directed health plans, too. These plans, their supporters argue, promise greater efficiency in reducing costs and raising quality. Currently, health care consumers lack the most basic information supplied by normal markets, most importantly, comparative pricing. Not only are consumers shielded from the full cost of their health insurance and health care by tax deductions and third-party payments, but it is also nearly impossible to compare the prices of the services offered by different physicians and hospitals. In addition, there are quality ratings for many products—automobiles, appliances, mutual funds—but little information about health outcomes achieved by different providers, pharmaceutical drugs, or medical devices. This lack of transparency in price and quality must be corrected somehow, as market reformers are right to insist.

Market reformers foresee tens of millions of choosy consumers as the remedy. Money talks, as the saying goes. If Americans spent more of their own money on health insurance and health care, then money would talk very clearly to consumers, providers, and insurers. The messages to consumers would be to demand price lists from providers and quality information from ratings companies; choose physicians and hospitals that provide the best value for the money; select insurance plans tailored to your own health needs, provider preferences, and chronic conditions, if any; and invest in wellness through better eating, more exercise, and fewer risky behaviors. Providers would be told to compete on the basis of price and outcomes for clinical care, pharmaceuticals, and medical devices; and build teams of physicians, nurses, pharmacists, and social workers to integrate care and pioneer cost-effective protocols, especially in such high-cost sectors as chronic disease and geriatrics. Insurers would be told to give consumers incentives to invest in personal wellness; partner with providers delivering high-value care; and offer a variety of policies and provider networks that target different health profiles, particularly for patients with chronic conditions where the largest cost savings might be recouped.

Behind all of these messages is the economic premise that consumers spend their limited money based on current market prices and their own preferences. Patients with high-deductible health plans would certainly get a bracing reckoning with health care prices. Purchasing health insurance directly, even with employer assistance or public subsidies, would make the personal costs of US health care much more transparent. Whether these consumer-directed plans can clarify consumers' actual health care preferences and make US health care more efficient is debatable, however, as I discuss in chapter 5.

MARKET ECONOMICS AND COMMUTATIVE JUSTICE

Market reformers have captured conservatives' minds and hearts because their economic and justice arguments fit hand in glove—a consistency that is sorely missing in the idea of health care as a private benefit as it is practiced in the United States. Claiming that "I own my health care benefits," even though other people have funded most of my Medicare bills, makes no sense to market reformers. Although they would never use the term "social," they do acknowledge that there would be some limited social sharing in risks and costs in the catastrophic care portion of consumer-directed health plans, just as there is with homeowner and automobile insurance policies. But the main point here is that a model of US health care in which consumers own the health insurance and health care services they pay for would be ruled not by distributive justice but by commutative justice.

For market reformers health care is not a good that Americans jointly produce, pay for, and use, the premise of distributive justice. Commutative justice does not start with shared goods and does not ask how shared goods are distributed among people. It looks exclusively to people's direct exchanges of private goods, declaring the transactions to be just if the contracting parties begin with adequate information, then voluntarily agree on the equivalence of the money and services being exchanged, and finally fulfill the terms of their contract. From the standpoint of commutative justice (also called justice in exchange), health care justice is the sum total of all of the voluntary transactions between consumers and providers and between consumers and insurers. Thus the people who buy their health care services directly and who purchase their insurance policy individually own these services and coverage by law and by right. By contrast, noncontributors have no justice claims whatsoever, whether on providers, insurers, or fellow citizens. Uncompensated care might be provided as charity, but not deserved as a right or guaranteed as a need. For market reformers free exchange means free exchange alone, without the complicating demands of desert and need added to the equation.

The market reformers' approach to health care reform centers on choice, quality, and cost, not the triad of access, quality, and cost that liberal reformers stress. Choice must be a leading value, the economic argument goes, because quality improvements and cost reductions follow from consumer demands and provider innovation. The expectation of financial reward is needed to motivate consumers to invest time and research in seeking high-value care. Financial reward also motivates providers to invest in the training and infrastructure to deliver better services. That is how market incentives work economically. Here it must be said, however, that an ethical notion of special desert in the form of social value still clings to this market economics. People who receive financial recompense through prudent consumption or innovative enterprise deserve their rewards as a matter of justice. In the words of health policy expert Robert Moffit of the conservative Heritage Foundation, "Those who make enormous contributions of time and labor in the system will be able to reap the just deserts of their efforts; their due."[37] To this way of thinking, the people who invest the most deserve to get more back, not simply because of their contracted property rights but also because other Americans will benefit as the predicted cost reductions and quality improvements they pioneered become more widely adopted. Ultimately, if costs drop far enough, there is the promise of expanded access for people currently priced out of the markets for health insurance and health care. Thus the value of access reenters the market reformers' vision as a hoped-for side effect, though not as a driving goal. Expanded access is the caboose parked several stations down the line, waiting to be hitched to the train powered by the engine of private choice.

Rep. Ryan's Medicare reform proposals make sense within the vision of health care as a private choice. On the economic side, unleashing an army of choosy senior citizens, some of the biggest health care spenders, could revolutionize US health care and possibly slow or drive down the cost spiral. On the justice side, payouts to seniors would be limited to their past contributions as there is no guaranteed right to health care beyond the financial commitments that individuals have made. Indeed, given the crystal clarity of the vision of justice behind the Ryan plan, his further proposal to reform Medicare only for Americans under age 55 smacks of deep unfairness and political calculation. The consistent justice that market reformers champion would include *all* current and future seniors to achieve the promised improvements sooner and to stop the injustice of excessive payouts now.

The language of health care as a private choice and the grammar of consumer-directed health care have made in-roads not only among conservative politicians, but also among the leadership of religious health care organizations. A minority of the interviewees in my study of religious health care providers embraced market reforms. They offered three supportive arguments, which I will call the arguments from nature, from efficiency, and from justice. The argument from nature claims that human beings are by nature rational utility-maximizers who calculate and take advantage of economic opportunities. This position was expressed by the chief executive officer of a medical group affiliated with an inner-city safety-net hospital. Describing their Medicaid patients, he noted that "the patients may be poor, but they are not stupid and fully understand economic tradeoffs." They may enroll their child in one Medicaid-managed care plan for the promotional deal of a free car seat, only to shift to another plan to take advantage of its introductory offers, disrupting the child's continuity of care. Or these patients may seek primary care at the hospital's emergency department over their designated primary care doctor at a visit rate of almost three to one, greatly inflating the cost of their care. These choices are rational in so far as they accomplish something the consumer values—obtaining goods the family needs in the first case, or saving time in the second. Yet they have unintended costs. In the medical director's words, "without steerage in benefit design, patients will always follow the path of least resistance which is often the most expensive" for society. The best benefit design, he argues, would be high-deductible health plans for patients at all income levels. Medicaid recipients would receive public vouchers that they can bank for future medical costs or possibly cash in to pay for other non–health care expenses if they did not use up their designated funds in a given year. The argument from nature reinforces the disciplinary side of market reform.

The argument from efficiency focuses on a different part of economics—not what people are by nature, but how they judge economic value by making tradeoffs. What economists call efficiency is based on consumer preferences, and purchasing decisions reveal those preferences. Economists learn what people prefer—and thus value relatively highly—not by surveying them about their stated priorities, but by observing what they buy. In other words, people do not put their money where their mouth is; they put their money where their preferences are. A chief operating officer at a Catholic hospital welcomes consumer-directed care for "putting more market forces at play," which "will be good for rationing and rationalizing health care." The rationing he envisions is self-rationing, for example, deciding to forgo an office visit for "the sniffles that you might have had checked out before." The rationalizing across the health care system would come from individuals taking the time with elective care to explore providers' prices and quality ratings. "When you sit there with a $5,000 deductible, you do say, 'Well, my joint replacement surgery, which is an elective and doesn't have to be done today, let me make the call. Let me see. Maybe the hospital will cut me a break.'" If enough health care consumers become price- and quality-conscious, then some of the burgeoning joint-replacement surgery centers will have to shut their doors, he predicts, having "a good impact on the cost of health care." Market reformers forecast that both the decisions to forego optional care and the cost reductions in elective care can achieve greater efficiencies in US health care.

The argument from justice undergirds the other two arguments for market reform. Most market reformers emphasize hard-nosed economic theory, and it is easy to focus on the practical claims about market discipline and consumer empowerment that are staples of the reform debate: (1) people want a free ride, so comprehensive health coverage guarantees overuse, and (2) health care markets will unleash wise consumers, helping to stretch health care dollars. But market reforms finally hang on the justice argument: People who pay for health coverage and health care services own them, innovators deserve a larger payback, and there is no justice obligation to people who cannot or will not pay, even if some provision may be made in the form of tax credits, public vouchers, or charity care. Acting on this vision of justice, opponents of the ACA took to offering up their wallets in protest, dramatizing their belief that the law would steal their hard-earned pay to cover the health care costs of lazy deadbeats.

The consistency of the market reformers' justice argument has made them the leading conservative voice in the reform debate. Their clear vision of justice, stripped of all distributive elements, cuts through the muddle of values that, in their judgment, compromises the oxymoron of private benefits. If health care and health insurance are "private," then private individuals should pay directly for the services and security that they themselves choose. If instead health care and health insurance are "benefits" that are collectively defined by third parties and paid out by group policies with no premium differentiation among people's health risks and health care costs, then the benefits are not private.

FROM PRIVATE BENEFIT TO PRIVATE CHOICE?

The language of private benefits has been and remains the dominant vocabulary in the United States. Its historical origins are firmly rooted in the old private practitioner model of American medicine and the unique employer-based health insurance system that emerged following World War II. Despite more than half a century of transformation in US health care, most notably the development of expensive transplant, oncology, diagnostic, pharmaceutical, and medical device technologies and the addition of massive public funding through Medicare and Medicaid, the language of private benefits has retained its moral hold on the public mind. One of its virtues has been its hybrid character, the very element that market reformers reject, which combines a "private" insistence on patient choice and personal responsibility with a societal expectation of health insurance as a "benefit" of employment and retirement. Private benefits is an umbrella term that has sheltered an assortment of values frequently in tension with one another. For Americans with guaranteed access to health care, these values have appeared to be in reasonable balance. For health care insiders, however, this semblance of working order has been maintained through repeated policy fixes that contradict each other and through perpetual cost-shifting that frustrates an accurate accounting of the price of health care services and the overall cost of US health care. I return in chapter 3 to review the policy fixes and financing mechanisms that have shored up the private benefits regime over the years. Here

I summarize the values implicit in the two languages of health care discussed above.

The vision of justice behind the private benefits idea is clear: People deserve their contracted benefits because, it is presumed, they have paid for them by working or by paying their Medicare taxes. Two leading values associated with this language—patient choice and personal responsibility—combine in the image of productive Americans selecting their own providers and acting responsibly on the best available medical advice. There is also the value of security in having comprehensive benefits guaranteed by an employer or backed by the US government in the case of Medicare. When health care is needed, anxiety is a frequent companion to sudden vulnerability. So while the private side of private benefits confirms personal choice and worth, the benefits side secures quality care for unexpected needs. The distributive principles of free exchange, desert, and need all appear to be in harmony.

The value of access has also been historically served by the private benefits approach. First employer-sponsored insurance and then Medicare greatly expanded access. In 2011, just over two hundred million Americans were covered through their employer, Medicare, or an individual policy.[38] The private benefits system in the US has even served the value of cost control to an extent. In comparison to individual insurance policies, the group plans run by employers and the federal government offer coverage at lower prices through larger risk pools and lower reimbursements. Combining choice and security, expanding access while reducing costs, what is not to love about the private benefits idea?

Simply put, the operating premise that people deserve their health benefits because they paid for them is now so at odds with the realities of US health care that it must be challenged through a transparency revolution. Starting with the value of choice, working Americans have little actual choice in their insurance options, with most employers offering no more than a few policies and increasingly only one type of plan.[39] The notion that personal responsibility pays the bills is belied by the fact that the majority of the uninsured live in working families. In addition, privately insured Americans pay hidden subsidies, estimated at $1,017 for a family policy in 2008, to cover the costs of uncompensated care for uninsured patients.[40] The value of security is in decline with the percentage of employers offering their workers an insurance plan dropping from 66 percent in 1999 down to 57 percent in 2013.[41] The steady increase in coinsurance costs and high deductibles further chips away at the security once afforded by comprehensive plans.

In assessing how well the value of access is being served, we must distinguish access from coverage. Tens of millions of uncovered American have access to US health care through the unsecured and expensive back door of emergency care and other publicly funded remedies such as community health centers. Uncovered access has personal and social costs, however. The 200 million Americans covered by private insurance and Medicare are plenty large enough as a voting block to protect the status quo of private benefits, but it is folly to leave out one in three Americans from the one funding rationale (private insurance and Medicare) that has broad legitimacy in this society. Prior to the ACA's Medicaid expansion in 2014, another 62 million people were covered through Medicaid and the State Children's Health Insurance Program.[42] The remaining 50 million Americans who receive treatment sporadically in hospital emergency departments and community health centers were covered by an array of hidden public-funding streams, inflated payments from private insurers and large firms, and charity care write-offs and cost-shifting by providers. The complexity of this backfilling of coverage gaps contributes to the skyrocketing cost of US health care. The extra bureaucracy required by funders and providers and the misallocation of resources toward the expense of emergency care and delayed treatment siphon off funds from affordable, quality health care.

It is reasonable to conclude that the language of private benefits is not delivering on its values. It persists largely because of historical inertia and because powerful groups are served by its inconsistencies. Specifically, this language supports justice claims to personal ownership and meritocratic social worth that are factually inaccurate and morally self-serving given all of the sharing in other people's risks and costs in US health care. The hypertrophy of this sense of personal ownership erases social responsibility for shared benefits. Arguably the sense of entitlement is greatest both in expense and in attitude among the senior recipients of Medicare, not among the low-income people who are covered by Medicaid or who receive free health care. Unfortunately, the demographics of electoral politics in the United States prevents this truth from being spoken out loud.

Market reformers aim to break the link between personal choice and shared benefits. Again their vision of justice is that people own the health care services and coverage for which they individually contract with providers and insurers. Market reformers champion the value of personal choice at all costs, but choice backed by the value of personal responsibility in paying for one's own health insurance and health care. Put into actual dollars (using 2012 data), the value of personal responsibility would cash out as follows. The average family of four with employer-sponsored insurance would pay the first $6,000 to $15,500 of their annual health care expenses (minus any employer contributions to a health savings account). If market reformers succeeded in redirecting employer-paid premiums into employee income, then working families would face annual costs of up to $16,500 to $26,000.[43] Bear in mind that the second scenario presupposes that employers convert their annual premium payments to employee income. In addition, average premium contributions might fall with the spread of consumer-directed health plans. Even so, the figures are eye-popping. This level of cost exposure would certainly promote the value of transparency as consumers confronted their actual health care spending. Greater transparency would alter the health care industry by making price lists available and increasing efforts to quantify the quality of care.

Besides responsibility and transparency, the other values of market reform are economic efficiency and personal liberty. In theory—and we have only theory to guide us because no other industrialized country relies on direct consumer-provider markets for health insurance and health care—the spending choices of sovereign consumers, many of whom would be paying the bulk of their annual health care bill, would spur innovative efforts to deliver health care more efficiently. Economic efficiency is a complex value, but two dynamics describe it. On the one hand, a perfectly competitive market tends toward lower prices and higher quality in the goods sold. On the other hand, the mix of products in the marketplace responds to what consumers value.

Starting with the first dynamic, if consumers purchase health care services directly from providers, then the providers should compete for consumer dollars by reducing prices on current services or improving quality through innovation. Market reformers argue that such competition will be revolutionary, particularly in the areas of medicine that have stubbornly high costs like chronic diseases. In order to attract patients who would now be paying the very high cost of their care, providers would have to break down the walls between specialists, pharmacists, and social workers and create the fully integrated care needed by some of the sickest and most expensive patients, such as diabetics.[44] The second dynamic, however, cuts in a very different direction. Providers will have incentives not only to seek out high-cost areas of care that serve people's needs but also to gear their facilities toward more profitable areas, including plastic surgery, boutique medicine, and other high-end services that respond to the preferences of the consumers with the deepest pockets. For market reformers it is paternalistic to deny consumers the choice of whatever health care they are willing to buy, as consumers are the best judge of their own health risks and needs.

It is important to distinguish these two dynamics of economic efficiency—the pressure to deliver lower-cost, higher-quality services and the pressure to cater to consumer value. Market reformers emphasize the promise of less expensive high-value care without acknowledging that consumer value can be a creature of marketing fads, fear, and deception.[45] Responsiveness to consumer choice is always a double-edged value.

Ultimately, personal liberty is the supreme value of the language of private choice. Other than the market values of responsibility, transparency, efficiency, and responsiveness, there are no other values besides liberty in this model because the politics of personal liberty precludes legislating social values. Gone are the values of security and access in the language of private benefits. Security and access might be achieved indirectly if the economic efficiencies promised by market reformers are sufficient to drive down costs, making quality health insurance and care affordable for more people. But the thrust of market reform is against socializing risks and costs—the mechanism that expanded access and security in the private benefits approach. Although largely ignored by the advocates of private benefits, all social mechanisms for sharing in one another's health risks and health care costs effectively tax some people to cover other people's health care expenses. For example, the ACA's popular provision against insurance denials for preexisting medical conditions is paid for by its controversial individual mandate. The fabric of US health care is cross-stitched by a great many of these social mechanisms, as will be detailed in chapter 3. For market reformers, replacing personal responsibility with social responsibility interferes with the market freedom of individuals who could otherwise choose what health insurance to purchase and what health care services they need.

Market reformers are correct that the language of private benefits has become practically incoherent. In rejecting it, they also reject such current structures of US health care as the tax favoritism for employer-sponsored insurance, the power of employers to dictate employee health benefits, the state regulation of private insurers' policies and rates, government mandates on covered treatments, public transfers of Medicaid dollars to the poor, and excessive Medicare payouts to the elderly. What is fundamentally rejected is the social sharing in one another's health risks and health care costs. Without publicly disavowing the language of health care as a private benefit, market reformers nevertheless judge it to be dangerously vague. It is too cozy with the social mechanisms that join Americans in paying for US health care. In making health care a private choice, market reformers seek to avoid what they view as costly inconsistencies that are antithetical to American liberty.

I opened this chapter with the three distributive principles of free exchange, desert, and need. As the name implies, market-driven reform turns on free exchange alone. Nevertheless, market reformers make tacit appeals to the other two principles. When consumers pay directly for their health insurance and most of the initial costs of their health care, the argument goes, they are at liberty to manage their own health needs, and they have the financial spur to act with dignity in taking responsibility for their health. Health care as a private choice thus puts the determination of need and the affirmation of desert in individuals' hands—assuming, of course, they can afford health insurance and health care on their own or, possibly, with the help of a tax credit for every taxpayer, a voucher for low-income earners, or a subsidized high-deductible health plan for the poor, as various market reformers have proposed.[46] This caveat, that upward of 100 million Americans might be unable to afford coverage and care, raises a critical question: Whose personal liberty is championed by the language of private choice?

In taking up the language of health care as a public right in the next chapter, I trace the religious values in the many denominational statements that favor a right to health care. In these religious voices for health care reform, we hear a different set of moral values and a very different account of Americans' freedom and the place of health care within it.

NOTES

1. Keehan et al., "National Health Spending Projections through 2020," 1595.
2. Walzer, *Spheres of Justice*, 6–7, 9, 21–26.
3. Krugman, "Health Care Realities."
4. Martin et al., "Growth in US Health Spending Remained Slow in 2010," 212.
5. Keehan et al., "National Health Spending Projections," 1602–4.
6. As a public insurance program, Medicare is not a private benefit. However, in this chapter I lump Medicare in with employer-sponsored insurance and individual insurance because that is how Americans tend to use the language of private benefits.
7. Rep. Ryan's Medicare proposals have evolved over the years. In 2011, he proposed that all Americans under age fifty-five would receive annual premium support of $8,000 to help purchase private insurance. Premium support was adjusted by age and health and dropped significantly for the top 6 percent of income earners. Subsequent plans included the option of using premium support for a private insurance plan or a public plan similar to current Medicare. See Kaiser Family Foundation, "Proposed Changes to Medicare."
8. The Medicare payroll tax covers only the hospital, skilled nursing, hospice, and home health care portion of Medicare (Part A). The physician services (Part B), private insurance plans (Part C), and prescription drug (Part D) portions of Medicare are funded through general tax revenues and individual premiums. Thus calculating people's payments into Medicare is more complex than adding up their Medicare taxes. See Barr, *Introduction to U.S. Health Policy*, 115–19.
9. This discussion of employer-sponsored insurance draws from Thomasson, "The Importance of Group Coverage"; and Helms, "Tax Policy and the History of the Health Insurance Industry."
10. To make Americans more conscious of health care spending, the ACA requires that employer-paid premiums and health savings contributions be stated on W-2 forms.

11. Herzlinger, "Diagnosis," 32.

12. Butler argues that workers with employer-sponsored insurance resist consumer-directed health plans for two misguided reasons: (1) their "incentive typically is for decisions to maximize the benefits they receive—seemingly enjoyed at someone else's expense—and not to maximize value for money," and (2) they interpret attempts to give them more control of their health care dollars as harmful "cost-shifting" ("A New Policy Framework," 23).

13. Tanner, *Bad Medicine*, 13. By lumping high-deductible health plans (HDHP) with flexible spending accounts (FSA), Tanner confuses the issue. HDHPs require consumers to meet an annual deductible, providing a kind of shock therapy to consumers' health care spending. FSAs are like tax-free piggy banks, allowing consumers to deduct their ordinary medical expenses. The ACA limits FSA set-asides to $2,500 and excludes some previously allowed items.

14. Kaiser Family Foundation, "Exhibit 8.4," *Employer Health Benefits 2012*.

15. Thomasson, "Importance of Group Coverage," 2.

16. Reinhardt, "Employer-Based Health Insurance," 338.

17. Kaiser Family Foundation, "The Uninsured and the Difference Health Insurance Makes" (2012).

18. Kaiser Family Foundation, "Exhibit 2.1," *Employer Health Benefits 2012*.

19. A comparison shows the tax advantages enjoyed by Americans with employer-based health insurance over those who are self-employed. Using 2006 figures, the tax benefits for a family with an $80,000 annual income differed as follows: $4,925 with the tax exclusion for employer-sponsored insurance, $1,127 with the medical expense tax deduction, and $2,339 with the self-employed health insurance deduction. See Kaiser Family Foundation, "Tax Subsidies for Health Insurance," 7, 12, 15.

20. Thomasson, "Importance of Group Coverage," 2.

21. Reinhardt, "Employer-Based Health Insurance," 339.

22. Steuerle and Rennane, "Social Security and Medicare Taxes and Benefits over a Lifetime," 2–3. The authors calculate the "lifetime value" of Medicare taxes by adding a 2 percent annual return (on top of inflation) to the value of Medicare payroll taxes.

23. Barr, *Introduction*, 172.

24. For the HEART Act, see http://thomas.loc.gov/cgi-bin/bdquery/z?d103:S1770 (accessed Aug. 10, 2012).

25. One analogy that has been used to challenge the ACA's constitutionality is the comparison between the government requiring individuals to purchase a health plan and the government requiring individuals to purchase broccoli for its antioxidant benefits. This reductio ad absurdum foresees no limits on federal powers to regulate interstate commerce in matters concerning Americans' health. See Federal District Judge Roger Vinson's ruling against the ACA: *State of Florida v. U.S. Department of Health and Human Services*, 46. For a rebuttal, see conservative legal scholar Charles Fried, "Testimony," 5.

26. Herzlinger uses a food analogy to illustrate how consumers lose choice and employers face escalating costs in the hypothetical case of "breakfast insurance" ("Why We Need Consumer-Driven Health Care," 61–69).

27. Herzlinger, "Why We Need," xxii, 77–78. See also Goodman, "Designing Health Insurance for the Information Age," 228–32.

28. Cannon and Tanner, *Healthy Competition*, 67–69.

29. Ibid., 71–72. Goldhill contrasts catastrophic homeowners' insurance and comprehensive health insurance in "The Health Benefits That Cut Your Pay."

30. Reinhardt, "Wanted," 1447.

31. Joint Committee on Taxation, "Background Materials for Senate Committee on Finance Roundtable on Health Care Financing," 2.

32. See Pauly, "Adverse Selection and Moral Hazard."

33. For a very different cooperative model of consumer empowerment in health care, see Pearson, Sabin, and Emanuel, *No Mission, No Margin*, 45–66.

34. Herzlinger, "Why We Need," 4–11.

35. Cannon and Tanner, *Healthy Competition*, 117–20.

36. Hawkins reviews state policies on infertility treatment coverage mandates, arguing that even the most comprehensive add little to average premiums ("Separating Fact from Fiction," 203, 214–18, 220–21).

37. Moffit, "Personal Freedom and Responsibility," 473.

38. Kaiser Family Foundation, "Health Insurance Coverage in America, 2011."

39. Eighty-two percent of all firms offering health coverage gave their employees a choice from only one type of plan in 2012. See Kaiser Family Foundation, "Exhibit 4.1," *Employer Health Benefits 2012*.

40. Families USA, *Hidden Health Tax*, 2.

41. Kaiser Family Foundation, "Exhibit 2.1," *Employer Health Benefits 2012*.

42. Kaiser Commission on Medicaid and the Uninsured, "Five Key Questions about Medicaid," 2.

43. I calculated the annual liability of a high-deductible health plan for a family of four as follows: 1) add 2012 average worker premium contributions of $3,720 to the minimum $2,400 deductible mandated by the IRS for a low end of just over $6,000, 2) with copay and coinsurance costs limited to a maximum of $11,900 (minus the $2,400 deductible), this adds $9,500 more, bringing the high end of out-of-pocket costs to $15,500, and 3) adding average employer premium contributions of $10,409 raises the total cost range up to $16,500 on the low end and $26,000 on the high end. See Kaiser Family Foundation, "Exhibit 6.5," *Employer Health Benefits 2012*.

44. Lovett, "Chronic Problems"; and Stone, "Improving Health and Reducing the Costs of Chronic Diseases."

45. Reinhart notes "the huge gap between the economist's and the layperson's use of the words *optimal* and *efficient*" ("Efficiency in Health Care," 988).

46. The 2008 Republican presidential nominee, John McCain, proposed eliminating all health insurance deductions in favor of universal tax credits of $2,500 for individuals and $5,000 for families. In 2008, Indiana's Healthy Indiana Plan created a publicly subsidized plan for low-income Hoosiers with a $1,100 deductible and required monthly contributions to a health savings account. See Roob and Verma, "Indiana: Health Care Reform amidst Clashing Values."

Chapter 2

Health Care as a Public Right

The religious community was incredibly powerful in bringing God into the discussion in the sense of what is our higher moral obligation to our fellow human beings and don't we have a responsibility to others? It was very important for the religious community to step in and hold the Governor and us accountable not to the industry, but to God, and to use those words that it's about all of us, not just some of us.

Member, Massachusetts Health Connector Board

THIS CHAPTER opens with an observation by a member of the Health Connector Board, the board charged with overseeing the 2006 Massachusetts health care reform law. In our interview this union leader described how religious activists successfully brought God into the Massachusetts debate. Through petition drives, demonstrations, canvassing, and other forms of advocacy, the members of the Greater Boston Interfaith Organization and their allies across the state made the case that God wants everyone to have affordable, quality health care. From the state officials calculating the cost of expanded coverage to the insurance, business, and hospital executives eyeing their bottom lines, all of the key players had to contend with the argument that health care reform must answer to the dignity and needs of all of God's children, not simply to the numbers of the experts or the interests of the powerful.

What if Christians, Jews, and other religious groups brought their religious values more fully into the national health care reform debate? This question may dismay some readers who think that religious advocates are all too willing to "bring God" into public discussions. Indeed, some of the sharpest disagreements among Americans revolve around religious values and health care. In particular, such "life" issues as abortion, assisted reproduction, embryonic stem cell research, the withdrawal of artificial nutrition and hydration, and assisted suicide have long been at the forefront of bioethical controversy.

These debates reinforce two familiar views of religion and American democracy. The first is that religious activists always support conservative causes. This expectation did not hold in Massachusetts. The loudest religious voices championed the reform law, and they have continued their lobbying efforts in the years since. A second view of religion and politics acknowledges the diversity of values upheld by Americans and therefore opposes allowing any one group's religious or moral values to govern public policy. As the Health Connector Board member observed, "You can take ideas and words and turn them right or turn them left depending on who's driving the little God-mobile." Her use of the word "little" was not meant to be dismissive. It reflects her sense of the narrow scope of religious community compared to the universal reach of public law. In other words, only the members of a particular religious group will embrace the values that they believe are authorized by God, whereas legislative decisions and executive orders about public policy must appeal to the values spoken by all Americans. Even religious liberals who see God's law as higher and more comprehensive than national laws often affirm that religious values can enter the political sphere only if the religious arguments are translatable into a common political language of secular values and principles.

This modesty has typified religious liberals' contributions to the health care reform debate. For the most part, liberal Christian and Jewish leaders have limited themselves to issuing repeated denominational statements in favor of universal coverage, usually under the banner of a right to health care for all. Americans remain largely unaware of this longstanding religious support for universal coverage because the denominational statements are rarely read by the public and their underlying religious values are quickly replaced by appeals to universal rights in public debates.

This chapter examines this body of denominational statements to clarify Americans' third moral language of health care—health care as a public right. I first draw out the parallels between religious and secular arguments for a universal right to health care. Then I delve into the commitments to human dignity in liberal religious arguments and their background social obligations of covenant and common good. This discussion points to areas of common ground across Christian and Jewish traditions and, potentially, among religious liberals and conservative Christians, too. Most importantly, although their visions of health care justice differ, Jews and Christians, religious liberals and conservatives, all consistently affirm that healing is a shared responsibility.

As in chapter 1, I evaluate the language of public rights using the three principles of distributive justice—free exchange, desert, and need. Here the free exchange of market reform gives way to the priorities of desert and need in people's benefiting from health care together. As the Health Connector Board member said, health care is "about all of us, not just some of us." Religious liberals argue that everyone living in the United States deserves health care as a matter of basic human dignity. Furthermore, religious liberals describe health needs in terms of healthy living and wholeness. As a result, the shared responsibilities of healing extend beyond life-saving care in times of crisis to encompass the duties of sustaining health in all of its forms (physical, mental, emotional, spiritual) and maintaining essential institutional and community supports.

Liberal Jews and Christians are committed to social inclusion and holistic health. Note that conservative Christians' advocacy around life issues also concerns social inclusion: To whom do we owe the duty of protecting life, however this norm is understood? For many secular liberals, it is the religious source of these competing social visions that makes them too narrow and exclusive a basis for democratic deliberation. While the social visions of religious groups no doubt fuel some of the flashpoints in American democracy, editing them out of public debates will not remove the underlying tensions from public life. On the contrary, I propose that hearing out the full range of religious values can inject a broader sense of social obligation into the national debate, balancing out the individualism behind the moral languages of private benefits and private choice.

LIBERAL DENOMINATIONAL STATEMENTS AND RIGHTS TO HEALTH CARE

For many decades mainline Protestant denominations, Catholic bishops, and Reform and Conservative rabbis have issued official statements calling for a universal right to health care. For example, the American Baptist Churches affirm "that health care should be viewed as a right, not a privilege, and that the basic goal for health care reform should be universal access to comprehensive benefits."[1] Quoting biblical verses on God's ultimate power to heal and Jesus Christ's healing ministry, the United Methodist Church claims "the promise of God." Methodist "Social Principles," they continue, "recognize that 'health care is a basic right' rather than a commodity available only to those with means, and recognize 'the role of governments in ensuring that each individual has access to those elements necessary to good health.'"[2] The United States Conference of Catholic Bishops (USCCB) grounds the "basic *human right*" to adequate health care on Pope John XXIII's 1963 statement in *Pacem in terris*: "Man has the right to live. He has the right to bodily integrity and to the means necessary for the proper development of life, particularly food, clothing, shelter, medical care, rest, and, finally, the necessary social services. In consequence, he has the right to be looked after in the event of ill-health."[3] Although Jewish statements are notably lighter on rights language, examples can be found here, too. Referring to its 1975 resolution on "Civil Rights," the National Federation of Temple Sisterhoods "reaffirm[ed] its commitment to universal access to health care as a national priority and call[ed] upon its United States affiliates to support legislation."[4] In 1976, the Reform movement's Central Conference of American Rabbis agreed that "all Americans should have the right to adequate health care."[5]

This sampling of denominational statements reflects the prevalence of liberal religious claims that health care is (1) a right for everyone not a privilege of wealth or family, (2) a basic right from government not a commodity in the marketplace, (3) a basic human right essential to a person's flourishing, and (4) a civil right to be guaranteed as a condition of equal citizenship.

Each rights claim responds to a different perceived problem. The first two focus on the system level, criticizing the unfair privileges and profits that some people derive from US health care. The second two concentrate on the personal level, denouncing the denial of people's full potential and moral equality in being excluded from secure access. The two levels of criticism coalesce in the anguish voiced across these statements over the growing disparity between the enormous wealth expended on US health care and the number of Americans without health coverage. Comparative data dramatize the disparity. In 2011, the United States spent 17.7 percent of gross domestic product on health care compared with other large developed countries, which spent between 11.6 percent (France) and 9.8 percent (United Kingdom) of their GDP. Those countries covered all of their citizens, whereas 50 million Americans lacked insurance coverage.[6]

This shocking gap between the expense of US health care and the lack of full coverage should give every American pause, including defenders of the superiority of US medicine and proponents of consumer liberty to spend as much one chooses on health care. For liberal Jews and Christians, this situation demonstrates the inadequacy of free exchange as the sole principle of health care justice. They claim instead that principles of desert and need must take priority in responding to the human dignity that all people have in being created in God's image.

An important point of connection for liberal Christians and Jews is that human dignity requires protecting human life and promoting human well-being. The dual significance of the dignity that flows from the *imago dei* (image of God) is clear in Catholic social thought. In their 1993 "Framework for Comprehensive Reform," the US Catholic bishops state: "Every person possesses an inherent dignity that must be deeply respected, and every person has the right and the responsibility to realize the fullness of that dignity."[7] This statement motivates two different rights claims at the heart of Catholic thinking about the common good. The appeal to "inherent dignity" motivates the right to life from the moment of conception. The appeal to "the fullness of that dignity" motivates the right to adequate health care. The two rights claims are often at war in American politics.

Duties, not rights, lead the way in Jewish readings of *b'tzelem Elohim* (human beings' "creation in God's image"). The primary appeal here is not to the rights that flow from human dignity, but to the Torah's *mitzvot* (commandments, good deeds), which require caring for sick, injured, and dying people because of their dignity. The Religious Action Center of Reform Judaism advocates the "teaching that individual human life is of infinite value and that the preservation of life supersedes almost all other considerations. We are constantly commanded 'not to stand idly by the blood of our neighbors.'"[8] Here the neighbor is anyone in need of life-saving care, as God's divine image is present in all people. What do one's bleeding neighbors deserve, according to the rabbis? They deserve excellent medical treatment and a ready response. The commitment to excellence is reflected in Jewish tradition in the high value accorded to using God's gifts of intelligence and wisdom for medical training and innovative research. The commitment to a ready response mandates community support for developing both curative and preventive medicine and for maintaining health care institutions to deliver them quickly. As noted by the United Synagogues of Conservative Judaism, "Talmudical academies included in their curriculum medical studies, and scholars, according to the Talmud, were forbidden to live in a community that did not boast a physician and a surgeon. . . . As the Talmud observed, a healthy body must come before a healthy soul."[9]

The ethics of health care implicit in these Catholic and Jewish accounts of human dignity is an ethics of living abundantly sustained by a covenantal community or common good.[10] It is a short step to concluding that basic human dignity and full human flourishing oblige a society to guarantee its members the health care they need. Restated in the secular moral language of health care as a public right, *as guaranteed access to health care is necessary to both positive liberty and social participation, basic fairness requires a right to health coverage.*

We can sort out the connections and disconnections between religious and secular arguments for a right to health care by reflecting on a statement by Martin Luther King Jr., often cited in liberal denominational statements. In

King's words, "Of all forms of inequality, injustice in health care is the most shocking and inhumane."[11] Inequalities in education, employment, and income limit people's ability to participate fully in their society, but lacking health care access can cut more deeply into one's person. To deny health care access is to ignore a common feature of human life, the shared vulnerability to illness and disability and the personal suffering and social debilitation that poor health causes. When access is unjustly denied, mercy stops short too. Instead of comforting intimacy with people's bodies, minds, and lives when health care is needed, there is a callous disregard for those bodies, minds, and lives when health care is denied.

Although King appeals to justice and mercy, justice suffices in secular liberal arguments for the right to health care. It is possible to encapsulate King's own advocacy of civil rights in a secular liberal vision of justice. From this perspective, liberty is a combination of negative liberties and positive liberties. As a negative liberty, a right to life guarantees protection against one's life being taken unjustly. As a positive liberty, it requires active support, partly in the form of necessary health care to maintain wellness and to avoid premature morbidity. Moreover, for King, democracy enshrines God's love for all people in a political system obligated to guarantee people's fair equality of opportunity to participate in and contribute to their society. Thus basic fairness justifies a universal right to health care as both a precondition for full social participation and a social return on one's contributions into the health care system. Any barrier to health care access is unjust in thwarting people's positive liberty, and it is unfair given that nearly every American pays into US health care somehow.

Missing from this secular liberal defense of a universal right to health care is the deeper sense of social belonging implicit in King's shock over the inhumanity of health care mercies denied. King's moral lens was not focused on society as a collection of individual rights claimants, each deserving his or her due legal protections and guarantees. He saw all Americans as being on a moral journey together. The covenantal motif of the People Israel journeying to the Promised Land is at the heart of King's appeals to the Exodus narrative.[12] As with Jewish covenantalism, the duty not to stand idly by one's neighbor's blood binds together a people making their way as a community living out God's commandments. The Catholic ideal of the common good likewise envisions the *telos*, or end, of a flourishing human life as achievable only in community with others.

In their 1986 pastoral letter *Economic Justice for All*, the US Catholic bishops declared, "The ultimate injustice is for a person or group to be treated actively or abandoned passively as if they were nonmembers of the human race." The bishops meant both the social exclusion of aborted fetuses denied the right to life and the marginalization of any person denied the right to health care. In the bishops' words, human rights protect against social exclusion and marginalization by guaranteeing "the *minimum levels of participation in the life of the human community for all persons.*"[13] Yet even the Catholic bishops and the nuns who sponsor Catholic health care organizations were unable to agree on how these human rights apply to the Affordable Care Act. The bishops found the ACA's prohibitions against public funding of abortion too loose to support the law's extension of health coverage. The sisters accepted the Obama administration's compromise language as adequate protection and warned against missing the historic opportunity to secure care for the poor and the vulnerable.[14] Their dispute underscores the challenges that religious advocates face in translating their values into public policy. Human dignity and common good may cohere seamlessly in Catholic human rights teaching. In the adversarial political deliberation of American democracy, with its myriad rights to life, property, privacy, and possibly health care, religious activists confront difficult balancing acts. Perhaps secular liberals are correct. The justice of balancing individual rights is complicated enough without adding in the competing ethical claims of the social bonds and communal mercies advocated by different religious groups.

CONSERVATIVE CHRISTIANS ON HEALTH CARE REFORM

The challenges of health care reform appear only greater if we consider the relatively few official statements published by conservative Christian denominations. In their statements conservative Christians accept the need to extend health care to uninsured Americans, but they strike a different balance between justice and mercy. During the debate over President Bill Clinton's health care reform plan, the Southern Baptist Convention issued a typical statement acknowledging "a need for revision in the health care delivery system in order to provide affordable care for all those in need." It also cited the Southern Baptists' history of health ministry through "the establishment of charitable hospitals and clinics." These acts of mercy are tempered, however, by the overriding justice claims that flow on the one hand from God's being "actively concerned and involved in all of life," and on the other from the "Baptist heritage of insistence on limited government."[15]

This vision of justice is not the market reformers' libertarian justice of individuals bound solely by the contracts they choose to make. It is an ethics of life centered in family and church, with the state supportive of and limited by these two primary spheres of community. The family secures the health care of most Americans through jobs with insurance. The church extends health care by founding charitable hospitals and clinics. In granting tax exemptions to covering employers and to religious health care nonprofits, the state plays its own limited role, helping to sustain the ordering of health care obligations in this conservative Christian vision of a decent society. This vision fits the outlines of US health care today, so it should be not surprising that it has theological resonance and political power for many Americans.

According to the Southern Baptist's 1994 statement, national health care reform threatens to disrupt this proper distribution of health care responsibilities among families, congregations, and businesses. It therefore jeopardizes a health care system that "most Americans enjoy" and "is the envy of the world." Far worse, from this perspective, a "government-controlled health care system" puts an ethics of life at risk. In concrete terms, public funding of health clinics in low-income neighborhoods and in public schools is seen as opening the door to federal support for abortion and ready access to contraceptives for teenagers. In addition, budget pressures from rising health care costs may lead to the rationing of care "on the basis of economic decisions rather than . . . on the basis of medical need."[16] In the debate over the ACA, conservative Christian objections followed the same template. The National Association of Evangelicals reaffirmed that abortion and euthanasia are unavoidable temptations for state power. Likewise, the need to protect personal health care decisions requires that any reform plan "maximize the creativity of the private sector while minimizing government control."[17]

It is easy to lose sight of the vision of health care justice behind religious statements like these. The Southern Baptist statement appears to be little more than a series of objections to health care reform at odds with its professed concern about the needs of the uninsured. It can even be read as a callous defense of health care privileges that invite other people's envy, usually considered to be a sin by Christians. Letting the politics obscure the theology, however, prevents a thorough grappling with competing ideas of health care justice.

This conservative Christian vision starts with God's blessing of life, understood to stretch from the gift of conception to a natural death—or in the evocative phrasing of Cardinal Joseph Bernardin, "along the spectrum from womb to tomb."[18] Each person also receives his or her gifts and talents, which include the grace of disability and disease. Conservative Christians fear that people with genetic abnormalities and terminal illnesses will have no value or protection in the state's utilitarian, people-crunching calculations of "reasonable" medical care. Turning from God's gift of life to God's ordering of family, church, economy, and state, conservative Christians promote the family responsibility of earning sufficient income and benefits through hard work, with the diligent receiving their just rewards. The poor can be assisted by the charitable offices of the church, supported by the tithing of the faithful.[19]

The theological imperatives of neighbor love and charity for the poor distinguish this vision of health care justice from the market reformers' embrace of economic competition and individual ownership. Failing to see those theological underpinnings denies the moral concerns that motivate conservative Christians. It also obscures the potential for common ground between religious liberals and religious conservatives. Both groups place the health care economy in a moral framework of God's intentions for health and healing. In other words, the market reformers' master image of paying one's way in the health care economy is replaced by a divine economy of God's gifts of life, in which God seeks health and healing for all people. The locus of health care justice shifts, too. The fairness of contracts voluntarily made by individuals gives way to the justice and mercy of covenants bound up with God's purposes. God's desire is healing for all human beings, and God enlists people in comforting and caring for sick, disabled, and dying people. Healing is a shared responsibility for God's followers.

Certainly the meaning of healing and the scope of shared responsibility differ across conservative and liberal theologies. The differences can be summed up as follows: *a conservative ethics of life centered in family and congregation* contrasted with *a liberal ethics of living abundantly out of a covenant or common good.*

For their part, conservatives affirm God's gift of life as an original bequest at conception. This gift commands protection of every human life regardless of the value judgments that other people may make about individual human lives in the abstract. Keeping health care decision making in the hands of a patient's near-and-dear is thus a very high priority, and it fits the family-centric ethics of life at the heart of conservative Christians' objections to a government takeover of US health care. For religious liberals, life's protection must be extended into a lifelong series of blessings in living well. The need to secure the positive freedom of healthy living broadens the scope of justice, adding the shared responsibilities of meeting one's covenantal duties as a health professional or community member and promoting mutual flourishing in a common good. As effective health care becomes widely available in a society, it must be extended to everyone with greater security than afforded by the occasional mercies of congregational charity and the limited justice of family responsibility. In a system as vast, complex, and expensive as US health care, the government becomes the ultimate guarantor of universal coverage.

Tracing the dividing lines between these two religious ethics increases the prospects for reasoned compromise. Acknowledging the competing visions of life's beginnings should motivate religious liberals to steer the ACA clear of abortion funding. Recognizing how many Americans are left uncovered by either family responsibility or congregational charity should motivate religious conservatives to support the ACA's Medicaid expansion and individual mandate. Understanding the personal nature of decisions about end-of-life care should motivate religious liberals and religious conservatives to seek responsible ways to inform patients of their options and support families in their decisions. If, instead, each group retreats to its principal rights claim, there will be little hope for finding ethical common ground or for making progress toward lasting health care reform.

TWO NOTIONS OF DESERT: RATIONING AND ECONOMIC QUEUING

To illustrate the discordant nature of the American political vocabulary of individual rights, this section explores how competing rights claims play out in the health care reform debate. Earlier I introduced the vision of justice behind the secular language of health care as a public right. Because guaranteed access to health care is necessary to positive liberty and social participation, basic fairness requires a right to health coverage. Restated in religious terms, *God's gift of human dignity and desire for human flourishing oblige a society to guarantee its members the health care they need.*

This vision of health care justice shines a spotlight on the pervasive health disparities in the United States. As the Catholic bishops observe, "The health care in our inner cities and some rural communities leads to Third World rates of infant mortality. The virtue of *solidarity* and our teaching on the *option for the poor* and the vulnerable require us to measure our health system in terms of how it affects the weak and disadvantaged."[20] The Presbyterian Church USA notes that "African Americans are twice as likely, and Hispanics three times as likely, as whites to be uninsured. . . . Almost one-third of all American Indians and Alaska Natives are uninsured, a rate almost as high as that for Hispanics."[21] There is ample data that a lack of coverage contributes to inadequate health care access and poor health outcomes.[22] For instance, in 2003, the mortality rate for African Americans was 30 percent higher than for white Americans, and the

African American infant mortality rate was 150 percent higher.[23] If God's gift of human dignity mandates the preservation and promotion of life through health care, then a lack of guaranteed access denies people the basic respect they deserve. The resulting geographic, racial, and ethnic disparities in people's health translate these inequities into full-fledged discrimination.

The language of health care as a private choice approaches health disparities differently. In fact, health disparities result from various factors, not limited to Americans' uneven health coverage and access to care. Large-scale social and environmental factors also significantly affect people's health, including education, employment, safety, housing, pollution, and discrimination.[24] Personal choices about eating, exercising, smoking, or using drugs also affect health outcomes. Although the public may be deeply concerned about health disparities, market reformers argue that there are limits to what can be done if the affected individuals do not first take personal responsibility for their health. Giving people economic incentives to take better care of their health is therefore a core principle of market reform.

These opposing views of the causes of health disparities reflect two competing notions of desert. If health care is a private choice, then desert means earned merit. If health care is a universal right, then desert means basic dignity. The different understandings of desert are even more pronounced in the divergent political power of the term "rationing" and a health care insider term that most Americans have never heard of, "economic queuing."

Rationing is the regulated allocation of resources according to a person's allotment. Unlike food and shelter, which could be rationed according to predictably uniform needs, there is no obviously reasonable ration of health care for each person in, say, a given year. As a result, rationing in health care is taken to mean the denial of care for economic rather than medical reasons. Rationing occurs when a treatment, procedure, or drug is medically indicated for a patient but either the payers (e.g., government and insurance companies) or the providers (e.g., hospitals and physicians) deny care because it is judged not to be cost-effective. Critics also charge rationing in cases of medical "futility," when physicians determine that curative treatment or invasive life support is no longer medically indicated for a dying patient.

Economic queuing takes place when people who have no insurance or inadequate insurance must stand in line for uncompensated or under-reimbursed health care. There are several causes. Because physicians are not legally required to accept Medicare, Medicaid, or uninsured patients, these groups of patients, especially in the Medicaid and "self-pay" (which, as one of my interviewees put it, typically means "no-pay") populations, face an under-supply of willing physicians. Furthermore, the free or reduced care provided by law in hospital emergency departments and community health centers is limited by resource constraints and by the large number of patients seeking services. Finally, some poor patients delay seeking care because even the discounted charges are unbearable. For all of these reasons, millions of people line up for care. Americans who have good health coverage frequently excoriate the waiting lists for elective surgery and diagnostic testing in other countries, while ignoring the lines of people waiting their turn for an array of uncovered but necessary treatments, procedures, and drugs in the United States.

A charge of rationing can kill legislation. This fact explains why the ACA is relatively light on cost-control measures: More coordinated efforts at cost control would have eroded legislative support for the bill. By contrast, economic queuing provokes little public reaction despite millions of Americans having firsthand knowledge of it, not to mention the tens of thousands of annual medical bankruptcies that result when people receive care but cannot pay afterward.[25] What accounts for the difference between the two terms' political power? Unlike health disparities, economic queuing cannot be dismissed as the result of personal irresponsibility. People waiting in the economic queue may be scrupulous with their health choices. They simply lack secure access to health care. In comparing rationing and economic queuing, then, we must look elsewhere to explain the terms' unequal political valence.

Angry complaints about a government takeover of US health care suggest one possible explanation. Rationing implies direct bureaucratic denial of care, while economic queuing, when noticed, is perceived as indirect systemic misfortune. With rationing there is a villainous bureaucrat. Economic queuing is a social reality caused by no one in particular. Nevertheless, once we probe beneath the surface differences—anger at bureaucracy versus resignation over economic hardship—both phenomena equally involve denials or delays of health care due to economic cost; the patient wants care that simply does not pay for providers to give it or for insurers to cover it.

To probe the real difference between the terms' political power, we have to unravel the rights claims bound up in each. When care is rationed, one of two rights claims is violated—a right to life or a property right. If, for example, a hospital ethics committee agrees that continuing acute care for an elderly person is futile, critics see a violation of the person's right to life. What gives the charge of rationing its moral impetus is this specter of rationing care to disabled, terminally ill, or dying patients. A different rights claim lies behind most people's fear that health care reform will limit their care options. This fear gives emotional resonance to the objection that countries with national health insurance have waiting lists and, therefore, it is assumed, substandard care. When critics denounce the prospect of having to wait for a magnetic resonance imaging (MRI) scan or a hip-replacement surgery, they are not appealing to a right to life. They are claiming a property right to health care services secured by their private insurance or Medicare entitlements. They are also presupposing their desert in the form of earned merit in having rights to services that other people lack. It is not that their needs are different from uninsured people's needs; only their property rights differ. This subtle slide from right to life to property right explains the moral power of rationing language. Waiting for an MRI to diagnose torn knee cartilage is not perceived as a mere inconvenience. It is felt to be a potential threat to life and a clear denial of the personal dignity that having justly deserved health benefits confirms.

Economic queuing may also provoke moral outrage when a right to life is at stake, as the periodic public outcry arises when states propose not to cover organ transplants for patients on Medicaid.[26] What is missing, however, is public anger that the everyday delays and denials of preventive, diagnostic, and chronic care for the uninsured and underinsured are attacks on human dignity. Rather, in the absence of property rights secured through private insurance or through Medicare, there is felt to be no justifiable claim of desert. Again, desert here means earned merit. The claim of desert as basic dignity falls on deaf ears, despite the conviction expressed by every liberal Jewish and Christian denomination that every person living in the United States deserves access to decent health care as a precondition for being able to contribute to this society and as a moral recognition of our shared vulnerability to illness and disability.

The principle of desert has two distinct meanings in how Americans talk about health care. At times it is an appeal to earned personal merit; at other times it is an appeal to basic human dignity. When the National Council of Churches of Christ calls health care access a civil right and criticizes efforts to "privatize and 'individualize' Medicare," they are wary of this slippage in meaning.[27] Individual rights sound like equal rights, but individual rights can protect either earned merit or basic dignity. In Rep. Ryan's original Medicare plan, most beneficiaries would have received the same level of premium support for private insurance (adjusted for age and health). This guaranteed voucher would afford the opportunity for the same property rights to health care services. If, however, seniors with limited means were left with only the minimal coverage that their voucher could buy, they would not have the same effective rights because wealthier seniors would also be able to afford supplemental insurance. Nevertheless, in the logic of market reform, poorer seniors with barebones policies would have what they deserve—in fact, more than they deserve because their Medicare tax payments likely were below average. They would, therefore, have no legitimate complaint if they must wait in the economic queue. Market reformers are correct that Medicare costs have to be controlled, but for liberal Jews and Christians, cost-control measures must conform to a health care system in which deserved care is a matter of basic dignity, not earned merit.

THE POLITICS OF ABSOLUTIST RIGHTS

The revealing contrast between the political power of the terms rationing and economic queuing reminds us that liberals are not alone in attaching rights claims to health care. Liberals claim a universal right to health care; conservative Christians appeal to the right to life. In addition, proponents of private choice defend personal property rights to health care. Thus liberals who argue for universal coverage are not so much bringing rights claims to the reform debate as they are contributing to the knot of competing rights.

This knotty situation is made more tangled by the political dynamics of rights language in the United States. When rights conflict, their competing claims can be mitigated by balancing rights in light of broader societal goals. The American political vocabulary of individual rights, however, is characterized by trickle-down absolutism. In other words, one rights claim assumes supreme importance, and other rights have standing only after the dominant rights claim has been absolutely met. From opposite ends of the political spectrum, pro-choice opponents of any restrictions on abortion and pro-life opponents of abortion in any circumstances both practice a trickle-down absolutism. No other rights claim can infringe the right to privacy on the one hand, or the right to life on the other.

Consider, in this light, the three rights claims discussed in the previous section—a right to life, a universal right to health care, and a property right to health care services. I have described how right-to-life claims are the lightning rod behind the term rationing, lending their moral force to personal property claims to health care. Religious liberals and religious conservatives have some disagreements about what is required and what is permissible in proper care of the dying.[28] For any patient seeking care, however, religious liberals rank protecting life higher than, or at least as highly as, promoting healthy living. That is, a universal right to health care is not meant to trump any patient's right to life. Instead, religious liberals put a universal right to decent health care before personal property rights to any and all covered services. That is the liberal trade-off: *a universal right to decent care versus individual property rights to all care.*

In declaring this universal right, however, liberals invite the cultural force of right-to-life politics into the national debate. Because only one right can claim priority in trickle-down absolutism, political opponents recast the liberal trade-off as a universal right to health care over a fundamental right to life for any human being. Thus, it is alleged, liberals are so concerned with providing all health care services to everyone that, as budget pressures inevitably rise, the government will sacrifice life-saving care for the most vulnerable who contribute the least to society. As a result, a false debate takes center stage—think "death panels." Former Alaska governor Sarah Palin directed this charge against a pro-posal originally introduced by her fellow Republican, Sen. Johnny Isakson (GA), that Medicare pay for voluntary consultations between patients and physicians about living wills, advance directives, and patients' options in end-of-life care. Providing senior citizens with this information serves patient autonomy and the right to make one's own treatment decisions. In a politicized environment of trickle-down absolutism, however, policies aimed at balancing several competing rights are easily derailed by absolutist assertions that personal liberty is under siege. In the process, national attention is deflected away from the central ques-tion in liberal arguments: how to balance a property right to comprehensive health care for some Americans with a right to decent health care for all Americans.

Given this knot of competing rights claims, we can see why there has been little common ground between religious liberals and religious conservatives. Conservative Christians have effectively provided moral cover to the libertarian argument that personal property rights to health care trump a universal right to decent health care. Despite calls for mercy in caring for people who lack ade-quate insurance, conservative Christians' arguments make the right to life and property rights to health care services the sole concerns of health care justice. Mercy is also called for in responding to the needs of the uninsured, but it is not where conservative activists and religious leaders direct their moral energies in the health care reform debate.

At this point we should distinguish between Catholic and conservative Prot-estant arguments. When the Catholic bishops rejected the ACA out of their concerns about abortion funding, they also affirmed a universal right to decent health care and criticized the ACA for excluding immigrants from the new state insurance exchanges and Medicaid expansion.[29] For the bishops, rights are arranged hierarchically in this order: right to life, universal right to decent care, and property rights to purchased services. Any conflicts among these rights claims must be adjudicated in light of the social priorities of the common good, which include the government's "moral function" of guaranteeing the basic human right to decent health care.[30]

In a conservative Protestant model of family responsibility and congregational charity, just claims to health care services are secured by earning one's health benefits, paying one's Medicare taxes, or purchasing one's own insurance and care. Health care justice inheres in providing services to people who have paid into the system, whose merit is earned. Outside of this domain of justice is charity care. Given the cost and complexity of US health care, however, such mercy has proven woefully inadequate to ensuring that health care is available as a matter of basic dignity. Each time right-to-life objections are raised against policies to cover uninsured Americans, the follow-up questions should be: How far does human dignity extend? Does the claim of human dignity apply only at the beginning and end of life, making the earned merit of personal property rights the sole protection at all other points in a person's life? It is hard to square religious conservatives' absolute claims on behalf of human dignity with this tacit embrace of the libertarian principle of desert as earned merit.

This blind spot is particularly apparent in the strong support for market reform among conservative Protestants. One of the least appreciated aspects of the health care reform debate is that the language of private choice limits absolute claims to health care services. Market reformers have not drawn attention to this part of their program. Instead, they stress the personal liberty of contracting one's own health coverage and health care services. Property rights to these purchases are guaranteed, but only within the limits of what an individual can afford or chooses to pay. In other words, consumer-directed health plans remove the expectation of access to any and all health care services, whether secured through private benefits or public rights. The limit on one's "right" to health care is set by the consumer's willingness to pay. Rationing is achieved through market choice.

Before adopting the private choice approach to cost control, Americans need to acknowledge the prospect that some patients may die because their consumer-directed health plan does not cover certain life-saving procedures. If health care justice inheres in paying one's way and choosing one's covered services, then this prospect follows as a logical possibility. Thus one curious omission from the national debate is that pro-life activists have not yet labeled consumer-directed health plans "death contracts." The parallels to the supposed "death panels" are striking. In each case the goal is to provide patients with information—about end-of-life care in the case of "death panels," and about the costs of care in the case of "death contracts." In both cases, too, the goal of providing the information is to enhance patients' ability to make choices—about which end-of-life care patients may wish to request or refuse and about which life-saving procedures they may decide are not worth the price of insurance. Why then is there no moral outrage against consumer-directed health plans among pro-life Protestants? The cultural bias in favor of personal liberty—and thus in favor of personal property rights to health care over a universal right to decent care—is a major factor. This bias, which is at odds with conservative Christians' professed commitments to human dignity and health care mercy, warrants soul searching by religious opponents of the Affordable Care Act.

HEALTH AND HEALING, NEEDS AND LIMITS

The national health care reform debate has been locked in political arm wrestling over individual rights. In addition to the question of how to rank individual rights, there is the matter of how to set limits on rights once established. Rights are not absolute in legal practice, but they tend to be in American political culture. In the case of health care, for example, the move to manage care through health maintenance organizations in the 1990s provoked an angry response from covered Americans. Soon there followed patients' bills of rights that pushed personal property rights to health care back toward the absolute. With health care costs rising at unsustainable rates, any argument for a universal right to health care must clarify how this right would be limited.

In fact, liberal denominational statements typically stipulate a rights claim that is universal but limited—for example, a right to "adequate health care,"[31] "adequate and affordable health care,"[32] or "basic health care."[33] Because the content of these narrower rights is not specified, however, we must seek guidance about how to limit and prioritize needs in these statements' religious models of health and healing. What we find is a tension between biblical mandates to heal any neighbor in need and the broader social obligations of covenant and common good.

Biblical mandates to heal have a profound sense of immediacy. Consider in this light the command "not to stand idly by the blood of our neighbors" (Lev. 19:16). This evocative phrase echoes with the justice of a direct obligation to tend to the needs of a person bleeding right before one's eyes. In Jewish tradition the urgency of this individual duty is so great that the mitzvah of saving a person from endangerment to human life (*pikuah nefesh*) supersedes all but three other duties. Traditionally, only the negative commandments of avoiding murder, idolatry, and adultery took precedence over the positive duty to heal. Every other mitzvah, including the obligation to rest on the Sabbath, must be suspended when the duty to heal is in play.[34] This simple model clearly puts priority on people's health care need in times of crisis, but it leaves important questions unanswered. Does health care justice demand only life-saving care? In what ways are people without medical skills obliged by health care justice?

To answer these questions, we must look beyond the biblical mandate to the covenantal ethics of Judaism. An arresting phrase from Jewish ethicist Elliot Dorff—"love your neighbor *and* yourself"—introduces the broad array and complex balancing of duties in Jewish tradition.[35] The rabbis of the Talmud observed that bodily life and health are required for individuals to be able to fulfill their duties to other people. We can see just how high a priority self-preservation has in a rabbinical discussion of two people traveling through a desert with only enough water to keep one of them alive. In Rabbi Akiva's classical ruling, since only one life can be saved, the life of the owner of the lone water flask takes precedence.[36] Turning from the extremity of this case to a broader health care ethics, the United Synagogues of Conservative Judaism extend the duty of self-preservation into personal stewardship of one's health: "In Deuteronomy God tells the Jewish people, 'take utmost care and watch yourselves scrupulously'" (Deut. 4:9). Maimonides, the twelfth-century synthesizer of *halakhah* (Jewish law), codified this passage as requiring both the positive duties of "regular exercise and seeking out proper medical care" and the negative duties of avoiding harmful food and drugs. Preserving health and wellness not only honors God's gift of life, but also allows one to fulfill one's covenantal obligations. Among the most important duties incumbent on healthy Jews is visiting and comforting the sick (*bikkur holim*).[37]

Although all Jews share in these individual obligations, Jewish ethics does not impose the same duties of healing on everyone, but divides them across different social roles. Clearly, the mitzvah of not standing idly by our neighbor's blood commands an active response from skilled physicians and nurses offering life-saving care. As human beings are co-creators with God in Jewish tradition, these professionals should also use their "understanding and ability" to develop a range of treatments, including the preventive and routine care necessary to maintaining bodily health.[38] Members of the community have active roles to play in support, too. Without communal funding, the medical infrastructure would not exist for training and research. Without a willing *tzedakah* (justice, financial support) for patients who cannot pay, caregivers would be unfairly burdened in providing free care, eroding their capacity to meet their other duties. Without individuals caring for themselves, undue financial burdens

would befall their fellow community members. In short, a whole series of covenantal obligations attaches to this central Jewish command.

This concatenation of spheres of covenantal responsibility can seem practically unlimited in its reach and demands. Yet there are two constraints. First, by
delineating responsibilities in distinct social spheres, this structured accounting
of duties allows any one group to argue that its obligations should be limited in
favor of another's. For example, physicians can set limits on their charity care
obligations. At the same time, if physicians pursued a research agenda focused
exclusively on life-saving therapies, they would fall short of the biblical mandate
of wellness and prevention. Poorer patients burdened by health care costs could
seek redress from the community on grounds of *tzedakah*. The community, for
its part, should be able to limit its duties to patients who disregard all personal
stewardship of their health.

Second, because rights derive from duties in Jewish tradition, there is no
absolutism of inherent rights, even if the primary duty of life-saving care is
nearly categorical. In Dorff's words, "If . . . the prime fact of my being is that I
have obligations, as it is in Judaism, then the burden of proof rests upon me to
demonstrate that I have a right against another person as a result of his or her
duties. My rights exist only to the extent that others have obligations to me, not
as an innate characteristic of my being."[39] The duty-centered nature of Jewish
ethics helps explain why Jewish denominational statements use the language of
rights infrequently. Because covenants are communal, individual rights cannot
be unlimited. They cannot be allowed to tax the community's capacity past its
own survival. Summing up, these two covenantal constraints—the structured
accounting of social duties and the ultimate limit on a community's duties—do
not specify exactly which health needs must be met. Instead, they identify
important social priorities to consider as the national debate increasingly turns
to the question of how to control costs.

A favorite liberal Christian model of biblical healing is the parable of the
Good Samaritan (Lk. 10:25–37). The United Church of Christ, for example,
takes Jesus's teaching about neighbor love as its model: "Through his exemplary
life we, as his followers today, are called to the ever-widening ministry of healing.
The familiar story of the Good Samaritan makes a direct case for universal access
to health care. We are reminded to love our neighbor, stop and touch the pain,
then assist in a caring manner to nurture the neighbor back to health and wholeness."[40] The biblical appeal is once again to a direct obligation on anyone who
finds him or herself facing a suffering neighbor. Here the mandate is not simply
to stop the bleeding of the person before one, but to restore any neighbor to
health and wholeness.

The intensely spiritual and holistic appeal of this call to restore the neighbor to health and wholeness distinguishes liberal Christian from liberal Jewish statements on health care justice. In most Christian statements health care responsibilities are doubly determined by the covenantal duties of justice and by the Gospel response of love.[41] The double source of moral obligation is clear in this rendering of the Good Samaritan parable, which telescopes out from the immediacy of stopping and touching the neighbor's pain to the civic duty of supporting universal access to health care for any neighbor (presumably in the United States). The distinction made here is not meant to echo Christian criticism of the Torah's "law" versus the Gospel's "grace." Jewish ethics joins personal visits to the sick with community support for neighbors in need. Compassion and mercy are central here, too. Rather, my aim is to highlight the more unbounded scope of health needs and healing responsibilities in liberal Christian statements.

Despite casting a broader net, Christian denominational statements have social priorities written into them, too. The American Baptist Churches' statement on "Health, Healing and Wholeness" equates health with *shalom*, which, the statement notes, is typically translated too narrowly as "peace." Shalom is instead "a dynamic condition of wholeness and fulfillment in every aspect of life: physical, mental and spiritual, as well as individual and communal."[42] This multifaceted understanding of health speaks to the many shortcomings of US health care that the United Church of Christ's "ever-widening ministry of healing" seeks to remedy. Specifically, lack of access to health care involves a series of reinforcing injustices: the refusal to care for people's bodies and minds and, adding insult to injury, the spiritual despair of social exclusion.[43] The health-as-wholeness model, by contrast, requires not only including the excluded in standard medical treatment but also covering mental health services and reaching beyond the walls of clinics and hospitals to address the social determinants of poor health, which can be especially severe in low-income neighborhoods.

Meeting this full range of health needs would certainly extend the responsibilities and likely add to the cost of US health care. This goal is only *likely* to add to system costs because redefining health as wholeness would prioritize redirecting resources from aggressive medical treatment in acute care facilities to supportive care in communities. Examples of community care might include the delivery of chronic disease management, obesity programs, and mental health services through community health centers. Although patient visits would be more frequent than an occasional trip to the emergency department, the cost of care for individual patients is likely to decline even as their health outcomes improve (see chapter 4).

Community care should not be restricted to health care facilities, however. As centers of pastoral care, moral authority, and community life, religious congregations offer the loving relationships and compassionate presence that people need to modify their behavior and sustain healthy changes, particularly congregants suffering from debilitating chronic diseases. Another area where congregations might make a salutary contribution is end-of-life medicine, one of the most expensive sectors in US health care. Although the American Baptist Churches identify health with holistic wellness, they add that health is "not a perfect or final state of being." Health must not become an idol that leaves us clinging to our physical survival or shunning the disabled and the chronically ill because they threaten a false ideal of health as freedom from illness and suffering.[44] Accepting illness, disability, and suffering as integral to human finitude and attending to mental, emotional, and spiritual health are fitting contributions for congregations. By practicing mutual care for one another's full range of health needs, congregants already ease the mental and spiritual suffering of the elderly and the dying. Congregations can also effect a broader cultural change, helping to redirect end-of-life care from heroic medicine aimed at battling illness toward personal wholeness experienced in a mutually supportive community committed to accepting death's time.

Two limiting priorities follow from this discussion. First, in the words of the director of ethics at a nationwide Catholic hospital system, the common good is an "infrastructure of well-being." This phrase joins the means of a massive health care infrastructure of hospitals, clinics, home care services, medical schools, research facilities, pharmaceutical and drug manufacturers, public health programs, and so forth, with the actual end of promoting well-being in people's lives. The infrastructure of well-being includes other social goods outside of health care, too—for example, safe housing, universal education, and a clean environment. If a shift toward health care in the community serves people's well-being while saving money for other essential social goods, then this social priority should govern public policies moving forward.

Second, congregations should reexamine the meaning of shared responsibilities for healing in their own traditions. In congregations committed to loving acceptance of all people, there is understandable resistance to practice healing as a form of scolding. Calling on people to measure up to a yardstick of prescribed behavior is not healing. That does not mean, however, that an invitation to health cannot be extended through wellness walks, community gardening, and other activities where healing is celebrated as a gift of community and a sign of hospitality. Parish nurses and church clinics can take this invitation one step farther into neighborhoods. Along with redirecting US health care from acute care toward community care, congregational responsiveness to a broader range of health needs may alleviate some of the cost burdens in the health care system. Regardless of their effect on cost control, however, such responsiveness is fully justified by God's call to mutual care.

CARING FOR HEALTH:
OUR SHARED ENDEAVOR

I take the heading of this section from the Evangelical Lutheran Church in America's "social statement" on "Caring for Health: Our Shared Endeavor." Notable about this statement is its lack of any mention of a right to health care. Through its twenty-three pages, there is only a passing reference to the biblical concern for the "rights of the needy" (Jer. 5:28) and an affirmation of "the right of individuals to be freely self-determining with regard to their own bodies and medical treatment decisions." The statement focuses on shared values not individual rights. The central values of life, stewardship, love, and justice are crystallized in the ethics of care in the statement's opening paragraph: "Caring for one's own health is a matter of human necessity and good stewardship. Caring for the health of others expresses both love for our neighbors and responsibility for a just society. As a personal and social responsibility, health care is a shared endeavor."[45]

This vision of health care as a shared endeavor is consonant with other Christian and Jewish denominational statements, with their covenantal duties of healing and call to health as wholeness in community. These broad social visions of covenant and common good tend to be supplanted, however, by two other priorities in religious liberals' statements on health care reform. First, biblical mandates to heal the neighbor in dire need reinforce the model of heroic medicine that already dominates US health care. Second, appeals for government action to restructure the health care system frequently displace congregational action in meeting shared responsibilities for healing.

Medical ethicist Larry Churchill has observed the individualistic and heroic overtones of the Good Samaritan parable. The moral action begins with the neighbor already in acute need. The Samaritan is anyone who happens upon the neighbor in dire necessity. The ethical mandate is to assume full responsibility for his or her health needs—"to love our neighbor, stop and touch the pain, then assist in a caring manner to nurture the neighbor back to health and wholeness." This direct person-to-person model is a powerful exhortation to neighborly love, but it also fits remarkably snugly into the one-on-one physician-patient clinical relationship that dominates the field of bioethics.[46] This direct person-to-person model of US health care is taken for granted by one of my interviewees, the director of ambulatory and outpatient services at a midwestern Catholic health system. In his words, "Good patient care *is* good community care." However attractive this truism may be in its stated commitment to care for each and every person's needs, it is not sufficient if it is taken to mean that good community care involves nothing more than the best medicine for each patient's health needs. Here community care is restricted to the clinical setting after a medical problem has presented itself, and the community's role is reduced to ensuring sufficient funding to extend the best medical care to everyone in need.

Bioethicists have focused primarily on individual decision making in the clinical setting by physicians and patients. The questions about distributive justice and the organization of US health care addressed in this book have garnered much less attention. Yet the more we focus our ethical lens on individual decisions about health care, the less we investigate surrounding "social practices," which in the words of Catholic ethicist Lisa Sowle Cahill, "favor the privileged and enable their free choices and access to resources [in ways that] carry a negative impact for global health patterns and the resources and choices of the poor."[47] To illustrate this problem in the US context, consider the following slogan: "No personalized medicine until every person has covered access to basic health care." The justice issue here is not simply access to a doctor's office or hospital. It is the astronomical price of cutting-edge therapies and niche medicines that puts them out of reach for almost anyone without the pooled funding of private or public insurance. It is the practice of steering research grants and honors to high-technology innovation, such as the genomics on which personalized medicine is based. It is the priority of discovering new life-saving cures for dying patients instead of learning to talk about death's inevitability and ensuring that people have life-sustaining companionship as their physical life fades. It is the competition among hospitals to purchase the latest technology to ensure that they have an ample base of admitting physicians to attract a steady stream of privately insured patients to cover the bills. All of these economic, social, and cultural pressures operate at the edges of the physician-patient relationship. Beginning the moral story with the patient in dire need attended by the heroic Good Samaritan doctor prevents Americans from asking if our collective march toward an ever-more-specialized and expensive acute care system is securing the health care we really want.

Religious liberals' denominational statements tend not to see research-funding priorities or capital investment in admitting physicians' happiness as justice issues. Even the high cost of health care is diagnosed as the result of the profit motive in US health care rather than the priority given to heroic medicine. Here we turn to the second priority that religious liberals fail to interrogate sufficiently in their denominational statements—the transfer of shared responsibilities for healing onto the government as the guarantor of individual rights and the agent of social reform.

For example, the United Church of Christ's healing ministry issues a call for a single-payer government health plan.[48] Other groups urge the federal government to use its regulatory oversight to streamline inefficiencies in the health insurance and health care industries, such as excessive administrative costs at private insurance companies; duplicate investments in expensive medical technology; financial incentives that reward acute and specialty medicine over wellness and prevention measures; and the expensive use of emergency departments to provide primary care for the uninsured.[49] Some statements go further than advocating regulatory efficiency. They summon federal power as a counterweight to the corporate power of private insurers, hospitals, pharmaceutical companies, and medical device manufacturers. Dubbed the "medical-insurance complex" by the Presbyterian Church USA, these forces take a deep and growing bite out of Americans' earning power and maintain a lock on their freedom to change jobs. Here the appeal to basic dignity behind the universal right to health care becomes a call for public redress for the powerless and the exploited, compelling the government to drive down health care prices and profits in an effort to protect personal freedom.[50]

This social justice critique of economic waste and corporate power in US health care is compelling. The prescription for reform should not blind us, however, to the implicit diagnosis of what ails US health care and how best to respond. The Good Samaritan parable is illustrative once again. As rendered by the United Church of Christ, the biblical mandate to "assist in a caring manner to nurture the neighbor back to health and wholeness" makes "a direct case for universal access to health care." Juxtaposing the response of neighbor love with a call for universal rights to health care gives personal urgency to supporting the requisite health policies. But an implicit tension must be acknowledged. Because the personal responsibility to care for each and every neighbor in need cannot, in fact, be met, personal responsibility as caregiver becomes civic responsibility as taxpayer. The focus remains individual obligation, but with the distance of voter advocacy for universal rights replacing the direct responsibilities for healing in liberal statements.

Three different approaches to defining social responsibilities and limiting health care costs run through religious liberals' denominational statements. First, there is the Jewish covenantal delineation of social priorities and spheres of obligation. Second, there is the Christian communal reclamation of health as wholeness in community, with congregations called upon to serve many health needs. Finally, there is the appeal to government to secure a universal right to health care services while restraining or reducing costs through mandated efficiencies and bargaining power.

In my judgment, religious liberals' arguments for health care reform have largely been ineffective because the embrace of government responsibility for health care rights has occluded the underlying Jewish and Christian visions of shared responsibilities for healing. Given the exceptionalist emphasis on personal liberty in American political culture, in the public debate the covenantal question of which duties we can afford to cover as a society is easily drowned out by the rights claims of individual Americans. Likewise, although mutual flourishing requires other social goods than health care, biblical mandates to heal, when translated into rights language, can leave the impression that each individual's every request for health care must ultimately be guaranteed by the government's legal obligations and taxpayer funds. An "ever-widening ministry" of healing can thus leap beyond a universal right to decent health care to an unlimited right to all health care without addressing some of the major causes of poor health. The impossible breadth of such a right reminds me of one of the chants used by the Affordable Care Act's advocates: "What do we want? Health care. When do we want it? Now!" Even as I echoed these words during a 2010 demonstration, a smile crossed my face as I imagined legions of physicians, nurses, technicians, and pharmacists taking our words literally and descending upon the crowd to inflict their care on each and every one of us.

Liberal denominational statements on health care do not seek anything so preposterous. People deserve needed care as a matter of human dignity, the statements argue, but mutual care extends beyond medical facilities to supportive communities. Some health needs—physical, emotional, mental, and spiritual—are better managed through personal choices, safe and satisfying work, improved social and environmental conditions, and a mature acceptance of life's finitude. Religious liberals balance a right to health care with calls for personal stewardship of one's health, for shared healing of other people's emotional, mental, and spiritual distress, and for public restraint in health care spending. When these arguments actually filter into the public debate, however, they are swept up in calls for an expansive and expensive individual right to health care, shorn of the keen appreciation for the social nature of US health care in liberal religious appeals to covenant and common good.

TOWARD A NEW CONSCIOUSNESS: HEALTH CARE AS A SOCIAL GOOD

As demonstrated in this chapter, religious liberals and religious conservatives both have social visions of health care justice and mercy. When the conversation turns to rights, however, the differences between their visions snap into focus. The priority of one rights claim tends to obscure all other moral commitments, lessening the prospects for common ground. The result is that both religious liberals and conservatives assume a defensive posture, becoming unwilling to seek positive balances between a right to life and a right to decent health care. The stalemate leaves a void that is filled by the most minimalist rights claim of all. Individual property ownership of health care services effectively trumps all other justice considerations in the health care reform debate.

Instead of appealing to rights, a more promising start would be to ask religious liberals and religious conservatives to discuss how they understand the shared responsibilities for healing in their faith traditions. An even more promising starting place would be to ask how they act on their respective commitments to human dignity and mutual care. I have argued in this chapter, however, that there is a strong tendency among conservative Christians to restrict the claims of human dignity to the beginning and ending of life and to confine responsibilities for mutual care to families, congregations, and religious hospitals. Yet many biblical examples of healing surpass these more immediate duties. Against family conventions of the time, the Moabitess Ruth chooses not return to her father's family upon her husband's death. Instead she cleaves to her widowed mother-in-law Naomi and returns her to wholeness in Bethlehem with the help of the community of women and a distant kinsman Boaz, who meet the fuller purpose of their covenanted duties. In story after story, Jesus reaches out and touches impure lepers, corpses, and the demon possessed, restoring them to health and a place in the community. These biblical models summon forth gestures of caring for and receiving care from one another as basic to our human dignity. They transpire against a background of inviolate community boundaries, making these gestures of mutual care all the more morally radical.

Given the biblical importance of *gestures* of mutual care, religious liberals, for their part, must accept that political arguments are not enough. Deeds are needed too, and they extend beyond advocating for a universal right to health care and paying taxes to fund it. Visiting and comforting people in their sickness, disability, and dying is a duty of healing for all of the religious denominations discussed above. Gestures of mutual care extend farther still. Catholic social thought commends the virtue of solidarity with the poor, and this solidarity must be socially enacted, not merely intellectual. Social solidarity has a different posture than intellectual solidarity. It is not the "aha moment" of moral reasoning or the conscious decision to contribute to a cause. Social solidarity requires physically turning to notice the people left out of health care, taking a stand alongside of them as people deserving care, and joining in efforts to change theirs into a situation one is willing to live with oneself. The examples of congregational care in the community, outlined in this chapter, manifest this spirit of social solidarity.

Religious liberals' invocations of mutual care, basic dignity, and solidarity with the needs of the poor are a quiet chorus behind the national debate, a counterpoint to the arguments that universal coverage is beyond America's reach because of the expense of health care or the threat of rationing. For liberal Jews and Christians, neither religious conservatives' priorities of family responsibility and congregational charity nor market reformers' priorities of consumer choice and provider innovation can supplant the shared task of caring for one another as if everyone's health mattered before God. Yet given how resistant Americans are to setting limits on rights through public policy, can religious liberals put their values of mutual care, basic dignity, and solidarity into operation without dramatically increasing the cost of US health care? As bioethicist Audrey Chapman has noted, liberal denominational statements are heavy on moral appeals to dignity and care, but light on economic considerations of efficiency, without which health care reform is unsustainable.[51]

Here we return to the fundamental challenge posed by market reformers. They accept our national unwillingness to set political priorities and limits in US health care. Indeed they embrace our distrust of building a health care system on shared values, and they propose the market as the liberty-preserving mechanism for controlling health care spending in a way that fits Americans' sense of their individual health care needs. Market reformers make one coherent justice claim: the sole guarantee of health care coverage and services is one's voluntary purchase of personal property rights, and any additional care is charity. This dichotomy between health care justice and health care charity is too stark for many, but not all, Americans to accept.

At a September 2011 Tea Party debate for Republican presidential hopefuls, Rep. Ron Paul (R-TX) affirmed this very distinction between health care charity and health care justice. He was asked if a healthy, thirty-year-old, single man with a good job who chose not to pay the premiums for his employer-sponsored health insurance should be allowed to die if he was struck by a terrible but curable illness. Although a few audience members cheered their support for allowing the man to die, Rep. Paul disagreed: "I practiced medicine before we had Medicaid, in the early 1960s, when I got out of medical school. I practiced at Santa Rosa Hospital in San Antonio, and the churches took care of them. We never turned anybody away from the hospitals." This answer distinguishes the justice of personal property rights to covered services from the charity of uncompensated care for the uninsured. It is consistent with then Dr. Paul's policy in his private practice of refusing government reimbursements for medical services, which he delivered as charity care instead. In the larger culture, Rep. Paul continued, the public safety net has habituated people into taking risks with their health care, knowing that other taxpayers will bail them out.[52]

Rep. Paul's response crystalizes the connections among the right to life, the mercies of charity care, and the salutary discipline of property rights in many conservatives' thinking. The right to life, he presumes, will always be honored by compassionate physicians and charitable hospitals. All other health care is best delivered through the marketplace. The problem with Rep. Paul's nostalgic anecdote is that it ignores the transformation of US health care not only in the overall cost of care but also in the variety and effectiveness of new treatments brought about, in part, through vast infusions of public funding for medical research and training and for public insurance programs, the proceeds of which most providers have been happy to accept.[53] Thus Rep. Paul's call for a return to old-fashioned values is at odds with the values built into US health care over the past half century. Religious nonprofit providers now direct their missions to more than charity alone, and public funding has invested heavily in health care quality and access. Looking ahead, chapter 3 details the range of shared values that nonprofit organizations and public policies have invested in US health care. By taking stock of these social investments of philanthropic service and public funding, we discover that US health care operates by a different rationale than any of the widely recognized languages of health care as a private benefit, private choice, or public right would lead us to expect. This book argues that Americans need to learn a new language of health care as a social good.

The language of health care as a social good recognizes that US health care works only if we are all in it together—benefiting together, contributing together, and, most importantly, working together to support the goals of health and wellness, while also setting priorities and limits to keep health care affordable. To return to the chapter's epigraph, the question today is whether health care is about all of us or some of us. Certainly, health care can be organized around each of us individually, as market reformers propose to do. It is difficult, however, to square this market-driven agenda with Jewish, Christian, and other

religious groups' commitments to healing as a shared responsibility. Congregations should add their own communal efforts to these social investments of
philanthropic service and public funding that have built shared values into US
health care. The more that religious groups step beyond their official statements
about individual rights and engage in practical actions of supporting and sustaining healthy communities, the more that US health care will manifest the
ideals of covenant and common good.

NOTES

1. American Baptist Churches, "Resolution on Health Care for All."
2. United Methodist Church, "Universal Health Care in the United States of
America."
3. United States Conference of Catholic Bishops (USCCB), "A Framework for
Comprehensive Reform."
4. National Federation of Temple Sisterhoods, "Universal Access to Health Care."
5. Central Conference of American Rabbis, "National Health Care Resolution."
6. Organisation for Economic Co-Operation and Development, "Total Health
Expenditures as Percent of Gross Domestic Product."
7. USCCB, "A Framework for Comprehensive Reform."
8. Religious Action Center of Reform Judaism, "Reform Judaism and Universal
Health Care."
9. Leadership Council of Conservative Judaism, "National Health Care."
10. Mackler's clear exposition of the shared norms of human dignity and justice in
Catholic and Jewish health care ethics incorporates Orthodox Judaism into this consensus as well. See Mackler, *Introduction to Jewish and Catholic Bioethics*, 191–96.
11. Martin Luther King Jr., "Presentation at the Second National Convention of the
Medical Committee for Human Rights," Chicago, Mar. 25, 1966, quoted in Advisory
Committee on Social Witness Policy, Presbyterian Church USA, "Resolution on Advocacy on Behalf of the Uninsured," 3.
12. King, *A Testament of Hope*, 136–38.
13. United States Catholic Bishops (USCB), *Economic Justice for All*, 18 (§77); italics
in the original.
14. Cooper, "Nuns Back Bill."
15. Southern Baptist Convention, "Resolution on Health Care Reform."
16. Ibid.
17. National Association of Evangelicals, "Health Care Reform."
18. Bernardin, *Consistent Ethic of Life*, 7.
19. Benne describes the ordering of family, church, economy, and state in a conservative Lutheran vision of a just society (*The Paradoxical Vision*, 82–89, 94–96). See also
National Association of Evangelicals, "For the Health of the Nation," 5–9.
20. USCCB, "A Framework for Comprehensive Reform."
21. Advisory Committee on Social Witness Policy, "Resolution on Advocacy on
Behalf of the Uninsured," 7.

22. Institute of Medicine, *America's Uninsured Crisis*, 57–83.

23. Williams, "Health and the Quality of Life of African Americans," 118. For other racial and ethnic health disparities, see Williams, "The Health of U.S. Racial and Ethnic Populations."

24. Daniels, *Just Health*, esp. 79–102.

25. One study cited medical bills as a factor in 57 percent of bankruptcies in 2007, the equivalent of over 160,000 filings (Himmelstein et al., "Medical Bankruptcy in the United States, 2007," 3). Even low estimates identify medical bills as a factor in tens of thousands of bankruptcy filings (Dranove and Millenson, "Medical Bankruptcy," w74–w83).

26. Sack, "Arizona Medicaid Cuts."

27. National Council of Churches of Christ, "Renewed Faith Community Universal Health Care Campaign."

28. See May, "The Burned," for a meditation on the conditions under which "life" may be so transformed by health crisis that refusing all medically indicated treatment becomes acceptable to a rational, competent adult. But this permissibility of refusing lifesaving treatment does not deny the right to life. For contrasting religious views on the ethics of dying, see Hamel and DuBose, *Must We Suffer Our Way to Death?*

29. George, "Universal Health Care."

30. USCB, *Economic Justice for All*, 27 (§122).

31. Central Conference of American Rabbis, "Resolution on Health Care"; Church of the Brethren, "Health Care in the U.S."; and USCCB, "A Framework for Comprehensive Reform."

32. Church Women United, "Resolution on Universal Health Care."

33. Episcopal Church USA, "Health Care Coverage for All."

34. Leadership Council of Conservative Judaism, "National Health Care."

35. Dorff, *Love Your Neighbor and Yourself*.

36. For an overview of and feminist response to rabbinical rulings on the distribution of scarce resources, see Zoloth, *Health Care and the Ethics of Encounter*, 160–231; and Zoloth-Dorfman, "An Ethics of Encounter." See also Dorff, "Am I My Brother's Keeper?"

37. Leadership Council of Conservative Judaism, "National Health Care."

38. Religious Action Center of Reform Judaism, "Reform Judaism and Universal Health Care."

39. Dorff, "Assisted Death," 143.

40. United Church of Christ, "An Urgent Call for Advocacy in Support for Health Care For All."

41. This observation that universal health coverage is doubly determined by justice and love in Christian traditions was pointed out by an anonymous reviewer of my article. See Craig, "Everyone at the Table."

42. American Baptist Churches, "Health, Healing and Wholeness."

43. United Church of Christ, "An Urgent Call for Advocacy in Support for Health Care for All."

44. American Baptist Churches, "Health, Healing and Wholeness."

45. Evangelical Lutheran Church in America, "Caring for Health," 1, 18, 22. The language of health care as a public right is also notably lacking from two documents by

the Episcopal Church: National Episcopal Health Ministries, *Healthy People, Healthy Church, Healthy Society*; and a report of the Standing Commission on Health, "Christians and the Formation of Public Policy about Health Care."

46. Churchill, *Rationing Health Care in America,* 36–37.

47. Cahill, *Theological Bioethics,* 3.

48. United Church of Christ, "An Urgent Call for Advocacy in Support for Health Care for All."

49. Los Angeles Council of Religious Leaders Health Care Task Force, "Theological Statement on Health Care," 6–7.

50. Advisory Committee on Social Witness Policy, "Resolution on Advocacy on Behalf of the Uninsured," 3.

51. Chapman, "Health Care Reform," 212–14.

52. Kaiser Health News, "Transcript."

53. Despite the large increase in physicians' salaries since the advent of Medicare and Medicaid, their average levels of charity care have dropped. See Kronick, "Valuing Charity," 994–96.

Chapter 3

Health Care as a Social Good

Going to have a conversation with the chair of the House Ways and Means Committee to talk about common good is nonsensical. So, from my perspective, there is a great deal of what I would call agenda-setting work that needs to be done, starting with community discussion and dialogue. People first have to understand that Medicare and Medicaid and public health care reform today is not just around poor people, but it's about all of us.

Government affairs director, West Coast Catholic health system

THE FIRST TWO CHAPTERS reviewed the three moral languages of US health care, detailing the values and visions of justice behind each one. This approach departs from standard assessments of the health care reform debate. Conservative market reformers and liberal rights advocates both start with a different question: What kind of good is health care? Conservatives tend to see health care as a private good, while liberals tend to view it as a public good. These empirical-sounding claims are rhetorically powerful, but they circumscribe the terms of the debate in ways that obscure the public-private partnerships that have built up US health care over many decades. This chapter argues for a different understanding of US health care: that it is a social good. The epigraph to this chapter underscores, however, the difficulty of changing how Americans talk and think about health care—not only in the halls of Congress, but also in the health care marketplace and in American culture more broadly.

As health policy expert Donald A. Barr observes, the organization of health care is not primarily an empirical question of economics. It is chiefly a matter of cultural values. "To understand a nation's health care system," he writes, "we must first understand the social and cultural norms and values around which that nation is organized."[1] Barr contrasts the approaches to health care in the United States and Canada, citing principles in each country's founding documents. Committed to "peace, order, and good government," Canadians have viewed health care as essential to the common good and made it a basic right. Celebrating individual rights to "life, liberty, and the pursuit of happiness," Americans have instead seen health care as a market commodity.[2]

To illustrate the market commodity model, Barr quotes from a *Wall Street Journal* opinion piece by Whole Foods cofounder John Mackey. "How can we say," asks Mackey, "that all people have more of an intrinsic right to health care than they have to food or shelter? Health care is a service that we all need, but just like food and shelter it is best provided through voluntary and mutually beneficial market exchanges. . . . This 'right' [to health care] has never existed in America."[3] Mackey's argument works on several levels. He combines a descriptive analogy about the presumed similarities among food, shelter, and health care with a historical observation and a normative claim that a right to health care never has and never should exist in the United States. Although I agree that there is no established right to health care in the United States, there are profound differences in how food, shelter, and health care are provided in this country. Like Mackey, most Americans do not appreciate the differences because they do not understand how US health care has been organized. Like both Mackey and Barr, Americans tend to see only two options—that health care is either a public good to be guaranteed as a basic right or a private good to be bought and sold as a market commodity.

This chapter develops an alternative. It explains how US health care has been organized as a social good, and it launches a normative argument, developed throughout the rest of the book, that national health care reform should build on this social good basis. The term social good needs introduction. Typically we use the moral term "good" as an adjective, not a noun. To say that something is *a good* in ethics is to recognize that it is something people seek in order to pursue their goals or meet their commitments. People desire all sorts of goods— for example, money, power, food, shelter, security, companionship. Such goods can be desirable in themselves or as a means to other goods. Health care is one of the means for maintaining and promoting the good of health, which helps people enjoy many other goods through their activities and relationships. A good becomes a *social good* when it is valued so highly by the members of a society that they share it and pay for it together through extensive and coordinated social investment. Other social goods include fire protection, universal public education, sewage systems, and water treatment facilities. Americans have decided that building and maintaining these social goods together is essential to making lives of opportunity and well-being available for everyone in our society.

Public spending is the most visible sign of social investment in US health care. In 2010, the government paid $1.2 trillion for insurance claims, veterans' health care, medical research and training, safety-net funding, public hospitals and clinics, public health programs, and other health care–related services.[4] Less obvious are the public values enshrined in the legislation authorizing this funding. In addition to public values, mission-driven health care nonprofits have contributed their religious and secular values to the operations, delivery, and financing of US health care. In these two ways, shared values have entered US health care through political deliberation about national health policy and through philanthropic investments by nonprofit organizations.

Once we begin to notice the social investments in US health care, the differences between the goods of food and health care emerge. Consider the comments of the chief financial officer of a Jewish hospital located in a poor area of a major city. When I asked him about the prospects for market reform, the CFO dismissed the notion that US health care works like a free market: "If someone comes to a grocery store, the grocery store doesn't have to give the person food. They will sell their food at a market rate or not at all. Our hospital and other hospitals don't have that choice; we have to provide a service, in some cases with no expectation of payment." The CFO readily acknowledges the compensation that his hospital receives through tax exemptions and safety-net funding. But these exemptions and funding streams fail to cover his hospital's losses on the uncompensated care that they are legally obliged to provide through their emergency department.

Other issues complicate the picture. In the world of grocery stores, there are the upscale vendors like Whole Foods and the down-market chains like Aldi. The economics of grocery stores keeps Mackey's chain from opening locations in Aldi neighborhoods, no matter how good a corporate citizen Whole Foods may be. It is possible, however, that a suburban hospital chain or an independent physician group could open a surgery center in the Jewish hospital's backyard. Despite widespread poverty there, the higher reimbursements that Medicare and Medicaid pay for surgical procedures could make this venture profitable so long as the new surgery center avoided serving uninsured patients by not providing an emergency room. Without additional laws requiring potential competitors to certify the need for a new facility, the safety-net hospital would lose its best business lines. Thus, for a variety of reasons—mandated emergency care, high reimbursements for procedures, and certificate of need laws, to name a few—health care does not operate like the market for food in the United States.

These examples barely scratch the surface of the complexity of US health care. Instead of dealing in vague analogies that obscure the issues, this chapter delves into the actual organization of US health care, first as recounted to me by administrators and caregivers at religious health care organizations and then through an overview of federal health policy since the 1940s. US health care is vast, expensive, and often convoluted. The current reality bears little resemblance to Mackey's imagined "voluntary and mutually beneficial market exchanges." In fact, market reformers largely concur. They recognize the many ways that health care does not operate as a market commodity, and they wish to dismantle the public policies that make US health care a social good.[5]

THE SOCIAL DIMENSIONS
OF US HEALTH CARE

To start, we need to introduce the primary social dimensions of US health care and their associated values. Jewish ethicist Laurie Zoloth describes health care as "necessarily social and socially necessary."[6] Unlike the essentials of food and shelter, a defining feature of health care is that it is provided in a social setting of caring for other people. Food and shelter can include this social element of direct care, too, as seen in the relationships that transpire at a farmers' market or a Habitat for Humanity build. These exceptions confirm the rule, however, that food and shelter are mostly provided across the impersonal distances of market exchange. In health care, if care is not part of the encounter between patient and caregiver, something vital has been lost. Without minimizing the importance of care as a clinical value, this chapter focuses on the organizational aspects of health care as a social good, which Americans largely do not recognize.

The first way that US health care is organized as a social good is the degree to which Americans pool health care costs and resources. This pooling includes the mechanism of private health insurance, which buys individuals financial security rather than health care services. In any given year, most privately insured Americans are not paying for their own health care or even their own actuarial risks if they are insured through an employer's group health plan. The comprehensive private health insurance policies that many working-age Americans have are a pooled, not a private, benefit, as discussed in chapter 1. Public insurance through Medicare, Medicaid, the Children's Health Insurance Program, and other government programs further extends this sharing of risks and costs. In addition, the public funding of medical research, training, and infrastructure has subsidized the building and maintenance of a vast health care industry that makes available an array of "miracle" treatments that otherwise would not exist. Every American is a potential beneficiary of procedures, therapies, drugs, and devices that would bankrupt all but the few were the costs of development and delivery not shared through the pooling mechanisms of private and public funding. This willingness to share in the expense of broad access to innovative health care helps explain why Americans have not yet rebelled against the greatly inflated costs that they face when compared to people in other developed countries.

The second social aspect of US health care is the unpredictable social lottery of health risks and needs. It is possible to go from a healthy, active life one day to a severely incapacitated life the next day, one that is dominated by medical routine and financial insecurity. The wincing pain and heartfelt sorrow that the healthy feel for people experiencing debilitating disease and disability signal a close identification with other people's suffering and force a recognition of our common vulnerability. Denying available care to people who cannot pay runs counter to these moral responses. It refuses fellow human beings a place in society and raises the prospect of one's own exclusion at the most vulnerable moments of one's life. Political slogans against providing care for immigrants are much easier to declare in the abstract than to enforce in person in the emergency department. Moreover, given the social risks of contagious diseases and other threats to public health, we recognize the shared benefits of treating individual cases and the shared harms of allowing them to fester. No matter how effective preventive care and public health measures become, our common vulnerability will remain, motivating the unspoken values of compassion and solidarity that are expressed in policies that fund research development of life-saving treatments like antiretroviral drugs or that guarantee health care access through emergency departments and community health centers.

The third social aspect of US health care shifts attention from the uncertainties of acute care to the predictably high costs of treating chronically ill and elderly patients and providing uncompensated care to the uninsured. These expenses consume a large proportion of US health care, particularly in the case of the chronically ill.[7] Critics of the rise in Medicare and Medicaid spending imply that it is possible to control these costs through voucher programs that leave people more to their own limited resources. But the costs of caring for elderly and chronically ill patients who lack adequate insurance will remain a social cost borne by the public. A majority of Americans will not tolerate policies that completely cut people off from health care, as evidenced by our current emergency care mandate. As a result, encouraging prevention and wellness and replacing emergency care with primary care to reduce shared costs are urgent social priorities that serve everyone's mutual interests. Finding other mechanisms for lowering US health care costs while preserving high standards of care is a social priority, too. Ironically, Americans espouse stewardship and efficiency in controlling costs, but they have proven unwilling to set limits on US health care. In the absence of effective tools for controlling costs, whether through free market means or government regulation, health care inflation will continue unabated. The accelerating pace will become unmanageable and erase any coverage gains produced by the Affordable Care Act.

Each of the social dimensions of US health care is supported by values that Americans share: *care* and *respect* in the clinical and hospital settings where patients are treated; *innovation* and *fairness* in the vast pooling of public and private financing; *compassion* and *solidarity* in public policies that help address our common vulnerability when catastrophic health needs strike; and *stewardship* and *efficiency* in the mostly unsuccessful efforts to control rising health care costs. With the encouragement of public policy, including tax exemptions for nonprofit hospitals, Americans built US health care as a social good by pooling shared resources and responding to common vulnerability. Today the question is whether to stay the course while finding better ways to manage costs or simply to abandon the social good of health care in an effort to control costs through market choice.

We can bring the economic and moral tradeoffs inherent in this question to life by listening in on an imagined conversation between two of my interviewees from two very different health care organizations. Religious nonprofit organizations are an excellent site for examining how such disparate values as innovation, efficiency, fairness, and compassion align with public policies and market competition. As these organizations strive to serve their mission while generating a sufficient margin to maintain and grow their operations, their leaders engage in an ongoing dialogue about the economics and the ethics of how to deliver health care. These dialogues combine realism about market competition with moral reflection on stated religious values.

COMMUNITY ACCOUNTABILITY
AND MARKET EFFICIENCY

The first person in this conversation is the government affairs director (quoted in the chapter's epigraph) of a Catholic hospital system on the west coast. Trained in Catholic social thought, he began working on health policy as a congressional aide in the 1970s. In our interview on the top floor of an airy art deco building, he addressed the challenges of translating religious values into political language. Looking back on his time in Washington, DC, he mused, "Going to have a conversation with the chair of the House Ways and Means

Committee to talk about common good is nonsensical." At its best, the aspiration of US politics is "enlightened self-interest." By contrast, he described health care nonprofits as "private institutions in pursuit of public good." Their purpose extends beyond the business of health care and the services they provide in their hospitals and clinics. At their core, he argued, they must have a "sense of accountability in connection with the community."

The second conversation partner is a physician-turned-chief executive officer of a medical group associated with the inner-city Jewish safety-net hospital. We met in a windowless conference room tucked away in a cramped warren of executive offices. Having worked most of his career at a for-profit physician-owned clinic, he described the business operations of for-profit and nonprofit health care as essentially the same: "It's just a question of what do you do with the profits. In a for-profit company you send them back to the shareholders. In a nonprofit company it's operating margin that gets plowed back into the business. But from a leadership perspective, there's not a big difference in running the day to day." In both types of organizations, revenues must equal or exceed costs, including the salaries of the physicians who work with uninsured patients. Good will never pays the bills.

Although the medical group CEO acknowledged the nonprofit commitment to community accountability, he did so ambivalently. Comparing his old for-profit clinic with the challenges of directing a safety-net hospital, he noted with some exasperation: "What we're terrible at doing here is prioritizing. In a for-profit market you've got to be very good at what you choose to do, and you don't lose a minute's sleep over what you choose not to do. In this [nonprofit] environment, you can't choose what not to do because it conflicts with the humanistic side of things. It conflicts with this idea that these people have no choice because they're uninsured." Two different priorities echo in these comments: accountability to the health needs of one's entire community and efficiency in producing high-quality services valued by one's patients. The values of community accountability and market efficiency frequently collide in US health care.

A clear example of this conflict can be observed in hospital emergency care. Given the central role that emergency departments play in the nation's health care safety net, my interviewees discussed the surrounding issues and policies at length. Although nonprofit hospitals have historically been expected to provide some charity care as a condition of their tax-exempt status, this expectation is now a legal obligation for every nonprofit and for-profit hospital with an emergency room (see chapter 4). The 1986 Emergency Medical Treatment and Active Labor Act requires hospitals with an emergency room to screen, stabilize, and transport any patient who presents with an emergent condition. In practice, emergency departments now provide basic treatment to nearly all people who turn up regardless of their condition's severity, though the long waits and the high expense are considerable barriers to using this back door into US health care.

This 1986 law is an attempt at legislating community accountability. It obligates hospitals to serve as the providers of last resort for patients who lack other options because they lack insurance. It is also highly inefficient in terms of cost and quality. Patients and hospitals incur crippling costs, which would be prohibitive of these services if not for the hospitals' charity care budgets and the government's safety-net funding. The words "charity care" and "safety net" are enough to turn off some Americans' empathy for community accountability entirely, as the government affairs director recounts from experience.

> People think it's all about somebody who should pull themselves up by their bootstraps. I've gotten more attention when I've said that one out of every ten children who's born in [one of our] hospitals goes home after day two and doesn't see a doctor. That's it. It's not the child's fault. Maybe their moms made a whole bunch of bad choices, but right now we've got a two-day-old child who doesn't have a doctor. Who's going to make sure that child gets twelve shots by the age of two? It's not going to be the emergency room doctor, and that's their only access point.

This anecdote breaks through the moral disengagement that the "responsibly" insured can feel toward the "irresponsibly" uninsured of their imagination. It shifts the response from scolding disregard toward empathetic dismay and, potentially, collective outrage. Why does a newborn deserve the lower-quality care that comes with sporadic visits to an emergency department, a poor substitute for the continuity of having a regular primary caregiver? Why should the public spend its tax dollars and private insurance premiums subsidizing more expensive, lower-quality emergency care? What kind of community accountability is this to uninsured patients and to the taxpaying public?

The medical group CEO would agree that using emergency care as a safety-net remedy inflicts discontinuous care on patients and social costs on the public. But he starts his analysis of the situation with market inefficiencies. Describing himself as "not a national health care guy, not an entitlement guy," he is nevertheless committed to a less expensive health care system that delivers quality care to the Medicaid and uninsured patients who make up 80 percent of the people served by his hospital and its affiliated clinics. Poor people have agency, too, he insists. Uninsured people make choices, and they act out of rational self-interest in weighing the costs and benefits of whatever health care options are available to them. The twenty-four-hour access of emergency care is a major draw for parents working multiple jobs. Despite the long waits, the one-stop convenience of an emergency department equipped with a full array of diagnostic machines can save time for people who lack ready transportation. Arguing that there is no effective financial disincentive for patients who cannot pay and cannot be dunned for not paying, he views the choice of expensive emergency care over a free visit to a primary clinic as rational, so long as only the costs of time are weighed against the benefits of treatment. When patients have to pay any part of the bill, the balance swings hard against this choice.

The medical group CEO applies the same economic calculus to the choices made by the doctors working in the clinics he oversees. In choosing lower pay than their suburban peers, the doctors were drawn by serving "a diverse patient population" and "the sense that they were getting credit in heaven for the good work that they were doing." But, the CEO observes with his business eye, "if you put [their numbers] under the microscope, they are making about what they are producing" because their patient volumes are lower on average. In other words, the doctors are not motivated solely by their moral commitment to community accountability. They trade lower pay for a lighter schedule, too.

As this CEO illustrates, economic incentives matter in US health care, and current incentives can lead to irrational outcomes. Subsidizing the primary care delivered in emergency departments wastes health care dollars. Low Medicaid reimbursements for physicians frustrate more effective and less expensive care out in the community. Thus market inefficiency undermines community accountability.

Looking at the data, there is, in fact, some debate over how much uninsured patients rely on emergency care. On the one hand, emergency care has been rising in general. From 1995 to 2008, there was an across-the-board increase in the use of emergency care in the United States, with privately insured patients accounting for most of the increase. On the other hand, uninsured patients rely disproportionately more on emergency departments than they do on primary care clinics or other health care providers. Over 25 percent of their doctor visits occur in emergency departments, compared to 7 percent for privately insured patients and 17 percent for Medicaid enrollees. Emergency care costs seven times a comparable primary care visit, so emergency visits add considerably to hospitals' charity care budgets, public subsidies for the uninsured, and the Medicaid program.[8] Perhaps the clearest evidence of overuse of emergency care is built into the structure of hospitals themselves. The old emergency *room* tucked away on the side of the building is now an emergency *department* looming at the front door. How has the United States arrived at the point where emergency care is a key tool in the nation's policy efforts to be accountable to unmet health needs even though it is an inefficient means for delivering quality care at a relatively low cost? Answering that question requires a review of the policies and values that hold the health care safety net in place.

HEALTH CARE SAFETY NET:
TORN OR TANGLED?

The image of a safety net is familiar in American politics. Despite disagreeing about its efficacy, liberals and conservatives view it in roughly the same individualistic terms. The safety net is meant to catch individuals who cannot grab enough of a hold on the economy to make a living for themselves and their families. For conservatives, the ideal safety net is springy, catching people's fall and bouncing them back up into the rough and tumble of the market economy. For liberals, people may need a longer rest on the safety net coupled with a ladder of social services to help overcome the structural disadvantages that the economically marginalized face in capitalist competition.

The component parts of the US health care safety net are a point of contention. When Medicare and Medicaid were created in 1965, both programs were considered part of the safety net. Today it is difficult to imagine that only 25 percent of elderly Americans had meaningful private hospital insurance two years prior to Medicare's passage.[9] In signing the law, President Lyndon Johnson declared, "No longer will older Americans be denied the healing miracle of modern medicine. No longer will illness crush and destroy the savings that they have so carefully put away over a lifetime."[10] Today, American seniors would probably be offended at the suggestion that they are protected by the nation's safety net. By contrast, the Medicaid program is generally viewed as "aid," as are the states' Children's Health Insurance Programs along with the other federal and state funding streams that help pay for uncompensated care.

A detailed accounting of government spending on uncompensated care challenges some of the political bromides on both sides of the health care reform debate. Liberals see the health care safety net as so badly torn that many people fall through the holes. Liberals' protests that uninsured patients are disenfranchised by US health care are harder to maintain, however, once we learn how far safety-net funding actually reaches. Conservatives criticize the health care safety net as a tangled mess that entraps people. Yet conservatives' insistence that government is the chief cause of the health care system's dysfunction begs the question of how tens of millions of Americans would receive care without the many strands of public policy woven into the safety net.

A shared assumption lies behind these stock appeals. They both assume that health care dollars should be linked to individual patients according to the services they use. Although both sides presuppose the fee-for-service model, they see the patient-dollar-service linkage running in opposite directions. Conservative market reformers want those dollars to *follow* the choices of individuals, with consumers buying their own insurance policies and much of their health care directly. In other words, health care is *my* choice. Liberal advocates of a right to health care want those dollars to *reach out* to any patient in need, with individual coverage guaranteed by law. In other words, health care is *my* right. Although the source of the dollars differs, the patient-dollar-service linkage is the same.

The problems arise, according to these standard arguments, when the linkage is broken. For conservatives, the more that bureaucrats interfere with the spending choices of consumers, the more that market inefficiencies creep into US health care. The biggest bureaucracy and thus the biggest offender, in their judgment, is the federal government. For liberals, the more that insurers and providers divert profits away from health care services, the less accountability there is to everyone in the community. To the extent that nonprofit providers act like for-profit companies in earning large margins, they add duplicity to their greed, their critics charge. These two lines of moral condemnation—"big government is the problem" and "health care is for people not for profits"— echo repeatedly in the reform debate.

Each line of criticism has some merit, which is why proponents on both sides can present their solution as the panacea for US health care. It is also true that health care dollars still largely follow individual patients and the tests, procedures, therapies, drugs, and devices that their physicians order. With patients viewing health care as "my choice" or "my right," and with physicians billing for "my services," US health care is locked into a "my mentality"—my benefits, my care, my doctor, my services, my fees. The result is an economic model that presses toward greater inputs and outputs, especially in high-need areas of chronic disease and high-profit areas of procedures, diagnostics, drugs, and devices. Far less attention is given to the health outcomes achieved and the organization of care itself. Despite the push in the 1990s to move away from fee-for-service payments for individual patients' care to the capitated payments that health maintenance organizations (HMOs) use to care for a group of enrollees, HMOs have lost almost half of their members since 1996.[11] Americans like their individual choices and their individual rights.

If we step back from idealized pictures of how health care dollars should be linked to individuals and consider how care is actually provided and paid for, a different vision of US health care comes into focus. The patient-dollar-service linkage breaks down most obviously in the uncompensated care provided to patients who cannot pay their bills and who receive discounted or free care as a result. The reason for the breakdown is simple: there are no individually assigned dollars from private insurers or public programs dedicated to caring for the one in six Americans who get lumped together as "the uninsured."

In 2008, the amount of uncompensated care for uninsured patients was estimated at $56 billion, with 62 percent of that care ($35 billion worth) provided in hospitals. Hospital administrators are understandably concerned about this heavy financial burden, though they are less vocal about the public funding that covers 80 percent of the cost.[12] Stepping back from the warring perspectives of individual choices versus individual rights requires us to step into the complexity of health economics and health policy, the messy world inhabited by hospital administrators. In this world there are numerous revenue streams flowing in the door; a variety of inpatient and outpatient service lines, each with different costs and margins; and a constant shuffling of money to cover the various services and to invest the capital to maintain and grow the entire operation.

Making matters more complex, health care reimbursement is inconsistent and cumbersome. In my interviews, one constant refrain was the problem of low reimbursements from government payers. The figures differed from location to location, but typical estimates put Medicare reimbursements at 80 to 90 cents on the dollar and Medicaid reimbursements at 35 cents on the dollar compared to hospital costs.[13] It should be stressed that private insurers also pay less than the charges billed by providers. Indeed, health care reimbursement in the United States is something of a great game of wink-wink and nod. Providers bill *charges* for their services—the first wink. Insurers adjust those charges down to estimated *costs*—the second wink. Then everyone nods approval that US health care operates through market competition. In the current situation providers can complain that they are forced to accept reimbursements that are too low. Private insurers can tout their efficiency in driving down costs for their members. Thus providers and insurers can both present themselves as performing heroic medicine in stewarding health care resources even as the costs of US health care outpace inflation nearly every year.

In fact, the only people who face full charges for their health care are uninsured patients with no third-party insurer, employer, or government agency negotiating reimbursement rates on their behalf. Any discounts they receive as uncompensated care are deducted from the original charges, not from the reduced costs that insurers pay. Uninsured patients do not get to play in the game of wink-wink and nod. Their double jeopardy of lacking insurance coverage and being billed full charges is one of the cruelest ironies in the (dis)organization of US health care.

From the perspective of hospital administrators, the relatively low reimbursements from Medicare and Medicaid create unfair shortfalls on care for individual patients. But there are two important caveats. First, although independent physicians may decide not to treat Medicare and Medicaid patients for reimbursement reasons, community hospitals cannot afford to be so choosy. A vice president for finance at a Catholic hospital notes that Medicare is its single biggest revenue source "by far." In 2010, Medicare and Medicaid accounted for 47 percent of total hospital spending, without which hospitals would be unable to pay their fixed costs.[14] Second, one group of hospital administrators welcomes both Medicare and Medicaid reimbursements, those who manage legally defined "safety net" hospitals (in cities) and "critical access" hospitals (in rural areas). The financial officer at the inner-city Jewish hospital exclaimed, "We love the Medicare patient here!" At a hospital where 80 percent of the patients are on Medicaid or are uninsured, Medicare's rates are very attractive. A nun who serves as mission director at an urban Catholic hospital system added, "Every hospital is going to have things that Medicare and Medicaid don't meet because the reimbursement might be low, though when we were losing money they were our best payers." Clearly, attitudes toward public reimbursement depend on how large an uninsured population a hospital serves; the grousing about public reimbursements is loudest at hospitals that perform the least uncompensated care. To make sense of this irony, we need to enter the hidden world of government funding for the safety net.

DSH PAYMENTS AND PUBLIC EQUITY

There should be a *Guide for the Perplexed* for US health policy to explain the countless acronyms used by health care insiders. In considering the question of why emergency care has been overused and what the alternatives are, two policies to understand are disproportionate share hospital (DSH) payments and federally qualified health centers (FQHCs).

The name of the first policy speaks to the value of equity written into US health policy. The "share" in the name is the share of uncompensated care borne by a hospital, and the implication is that every hospital should perform its fair share. This point is doubly important. First, there is a public expectation that hospitals will care for patients who lack adequate insurance. In other words, the value of solidarity is a social norm backed by federal law. Second, for hospitals assuming a disproportionate financial burden, supplemental payments are considered their due. Notice that justice, not charity, is the governing framework here. Burdened hospitals deserve this supplemental support as a matter of justice because they are providing more of the uncompensated care that the public and policymakers demand.

A commitment to broad-based equity was written into the 1981 law authorizing DSH payments. Equity was to be pursued at the state and federal levels and by hospitals themselves. The original policy encouraged states to charge all of their hospitals an annual assessment that the federal government would more than match. Payments would then flow back to burdened hospitals based on their levels of uncompensated care. In practice, some states manipulated this system by charging hospitals very high assessments to reap an even larger match from the federal government before effectively returning much of the initial assessments to the originating hospitals. The result was a wash for many hospitals and a relatively large pot of federal money for the state to distribute to its safety-net and critical-access hospitals. Although Congress subsequently ended this practice, the funding disparities became a permanent part of the DSH payment structure, allowing some states to recoup more than four times the national average for per capita DSH payments.[15] Thus, interstate inequities crept into a policy designed to promote solidarity in the health care system and equity among hospitals. Policy distortions like these can make even ardent proponents of a strong government role in health care want to throw a wrench into the entire health policy machine.

Despite the policy's shortcomings, DSH payments have been one of the mainstays of the health care safety net. In 2010, the federal government contributed $22 billion in Medicaid and Medicare DSH payments.[16] States add their own funds, generating significant supplements that have helped keep hospital doors open in inner-city and rural communities. The chief executive officer of the Jewish safety-net hospital stressed the importance of equity in a fragmented system and competitive economic environment. He related the story of two nearby hospitals, the first a Catholic safety-net hospital that was closing and the other a historically Protestant system that had converted an acute care hospital into a long-term care facility. According to the Jewish hospital CEO, the Catholic system claimed they "didn't know how to do" an inner-city hospital. The other hospital converted its services to offer a single service line funded by Medicare's relatively high reimbursements and closed an emergency room that served as a portal for uninsured patients. In the wake of this conversion, the Jewish hospital experienced a 12.5 percent increase (a thousand visits per month) at their emergency department, of which 60 percent were uninsured. In the CEO's words, "They got out of the [safety-net] business to become just a Medicare provider, and it ultimately punished us."

What happens to community accountability when one nonprofit leaves safety-net care for business reasons? Who will treat the patients left behind, and how will those providers shoulder the burden? These questions have broad applicability. In recent decades all across the country, US health care has seen the elimination of unprofitable service lines and the relocation of providers to the suburbs. Although an imperfect and incomplete remedy, DSH payments have nevertheless helped avoid the hollowing out of health care from inner cities and rural areas.

Market reformers would draw different lessons here. They would argue that the efforts of policymakers to build shared values into US health care—equity through DSH payments and stewardship through Medicare and Medicaid price controls—create perverse economic incentives at odds with policy goals. In the case of the Protestant hospital's conversion, it was the government's reimbursement rates that led them to shift to more profitable services. An immediate result was higher DSH payments flowing to the increasingly burdened Jewish hospital. How well, then, are the values of equity and stewardship being served? For market reformers the answer is clear. Public policies frustrate the "shared values" they ostensibly serve. It is better, therefore, to embrace market efficiency across the board, eliminating government price controls, halting DSH payments, and providing low-income Americans with vouchers and health saving accounts to buy their own insurance and services. Indeed community accountability to poorer patients and to taxpayers might be achieved by closing an expensive community hospital and steering its former patients away from emergency care and toward quality primary care delivered in less costly clinics—assuming, of course, that reliable sources of care can be found. That is the purpose of federally qualified health centers.

FQHCs AND SHARED RESPONSIBILITY

The sense that intractable divisions separate liberals and conservatives on health policy is belied by the historically bipartisan support for federally qualified health centers, known in ordinary language as community health centers. The FQHC category encompasses a variety of health centers that provide primary care to migrant workers, homeless people, Native Americans, and uninsured and underinsured people who live in urban and rural medically underserved areas (MUAs) or belong to medically underserved populations (MUPs). Consolidated into a single program under President Bill Clinton in 1996, funding for FQHCs jumped under President George W. Bush's Health Centers Initiative and President Barack Obama's Affordable Care Act. In 2010, over 19 million patients were seen at the more than six thousand community health center locations. Of those, 62 percent were members of a minority group (most often Hispanic), and three-quarters were either uninsured (37 percent) or on Medicaid (38 percent).[17]

Despite bipartisan support for FQHCs, the medical group CEO from above describes the centers as "a Republican solution for care of the underserved" because the policy aim is to correct the economic disincentives that physicians face when working in urban and rural health care markets. Here we arrive at a fundamental criticism that conservatives direct at Medicare and Medicaid. Because these programs reimburse physicians and hospitals at below-market rates, their critics allege that they create a host of irrational outcomes. Particularly with Medicaid, substandard payments deter physicians from caring for low-income patients in primary care settings. The medical group CEO cited an average Medicaid reimbursement of only $35 for a primary care office visit at one of his network's affiliated clinics, compared to $120 paid by private insurers to a facility in the suburbs. Although the reimbursement caps are meant to curb costs, the policy is doubly inefficient, he argues, first in the government's initial refusal to pay physicians' market rates, and second in the eventual high costs of the emergency care that patients turn to instead. FQHC economics shifts this pricing structure. The federal government bumps Medicaid payments up to the market rate. The quid pro quo is that the health centers accept all comers, with uninsured patients assessed a percentage of their fee on a sliding scale.[18] A similar program supplements the reimbursements for qualifying Medicare patients who use FQHCs.

In 2010, the total revenue of community health centers was $12.7 billion, including $9.8 billion from federal, state, and local governments.[19] Although accounting for less than 1 percent of public spending on health care, community health centers have become a mainstay of the safety net for poorer Americans and immigrants. Health centers do not offer straight charity care, as free clinics do. Instead, costs are shared across a range of payers, including the patients themselves, foundations, donors, and private insurers, with the bulk of the funding provided by taxpayers.

A Jewish physician at a Catholic hospital in a smaller city in the Pacific Northwest describes the situation that led him to found a community health center: "We saw a lot of primary care business in the emergency department, but we didn't see most of the people that needed primary care because it wasn't an emergency, and they'd rather not bother the emergency department. You find that this is a very stoic population." To staff the health center, they hired physician assistants and nurse practitioners, as employed physicians would have been too expensive and volunteer physicians too difficult to schedule. They partnered with three teaching hospitals to ensure a high quality of care and to train new practitioners in community care. To raise the half-million dollars needed to refurbish and equip the storefront clinic, they turned to the community. Local physicians, a Lions Club, a car dealership, the doctor's synagogue, and others donated over one million dollars. Within two years and with FQHC funding for its Medicaid patients, the health center was, in the words of the founding physician, "beginning to be self-supporting. But it's not equal health care. We can't, for instance, get all the specialty care we need." This doctor, who sees his Reform Jewish social justice orientation as perfectly in keeping with the values of his Catholic hospital, declared: "When all sin is evaporated from the earth, the Messiah will come. Be that as it may, until that time, I think the purpose of religious organizations, faith-based organizations, or service organizations like the Red Cross, the purpose is to see where society is failing and to fill those gaps. I see myself as a cork in the dike."

This story evokes conservative values of individual initiative, local self-help, and private charity. It should be noted, however, that the founding physician would much prefer to have some type of a "national health system" as found in every other industrialized country. Setting aside his wish for a more active government role, which he predicts would provide quality care to all Americans at a lower cost, it is important to acknowledge that this "private" effort at community accountability would not have succeeded in the absence of FQHC policy. To borrow an image from the Catholic government affairs director, the federal government's role in US health care is so extensive that even the slightest shift in the rudder of public policy alters the course of the entire ship, which he dubbed the USS *Health Care*. This navigational influence certainly applies to FQHC policy as the number of people served by community health centers doubled between 2001 and 2010. That total promises to more than double again as the ACA's expanded coverage requires additional sites for providing health care, particularly in underserved areas.

USS *HEALTH CARE*: SOCIAL PRIORITIES AND SOCIAL STRUCTURES

To extend the metaphor, a ship requires more than the cabins where passengers sleep and the meal, exercise, and entertainment facilities where they satisfy needs. For many Americans, however, health care is nothing more than the private clinics, hospitals, pharmacies, and drug and device manufacturers that dominate the one-on-one model of care in the physician-patient relationship. The patient sees the doctor, and the doctor orders the services and bills the insurance company. Unhappy patients can change their doctors or request better drugs. Unhappy doctors can refuse to treat patients whose bills are not fully paid due to poor insurance or no insurance. Conservative market reformers propose a theoretically elegant solution to the problems of rising health care costs and the irrational reliance on emergency care: By giving passengers the full bill for their accommodations, fewer of them will request first class. By guaranteeing doctors market prices for their services, more of them will choose to work on the lower decks, serving patients who might otherwise go to emergency departments. According to this view, reducing costs and caring for low-income Americans are both a matter of getting the economic incentives right. But this solution ignores the many other supports that have to be in place for care to reach these patients.

For example, the supply of primary care physicians and nurse practitioners willing to work in community health centers remains too low even with FQHC supplements. Another federal policy, the National Health Service Corps, reduces the gap through scholarships and loan forgiveness for health professionals who commit to work in underserved areas. The ACA dedicated an additional $1.5 billion from 2010 to 2015 to the corps' regular funding, and the number of participating clinicians recently tripled to nearly 10,000.[20] The location of health care services is also a problem, as almost all of the recent growth in the health industry has occurred in affluent suburbs. Without government assistance, it is difficult to obtain the capital for new construction and to recoup investment in poorer communities. With this in mind, the 2009 stimulus, the American Recovery and Reinvestment Act, allocated $2 billion to build and equip community health centers, and the ACA increased capital funding another $12 billion over five years.[21]

One clear social priority of US health policy is the commitment to provide a modicum of care for people without insurance, however uninviting the conditions and however onerous the billing practices may be. Without understanding how the values of equity and shared responsibility are written into DSH payments and FQHC funding, Americans may assume that the need for uncompensated care is minimal and easily met by the private charity of physicians and hospitals. On the contrary, uncompensated care demonstrates how dependent this part of US health care is on a social commitment to sharing in other people's health risks and health care costs.[22] Federal programs have been the catalyst for state and local governments, nonprofit providers, taxpayers, foundations, and donors to support legislated social priorities and to cooperate through the social structures of public policy. Even the current limited opportunities for uncompensated care require social investments of government funding met by social investments of philanthropic initiative by many different stakeholders. Such joint efforts provide an example of how health care is organized as a social good in the United States.

Market reformers argue that US health care must be saved by the "my" mentality that many Americans assume defines health care operations and financing. The problem with focusing exclusively on market efficiency, as if getting the incentives right would fill all of the cracks and fissures in US health care, is that it ignores all of the health policies that support the structure and steer the course of the ship. Conservatives argue that the supporting policy structures and directives should be dismantled in favor of vouchers for low- and moderate-income Americans to use as health care consumers. Like any other person booking passage, these Americans would take their place in the direct markets between physicians and patients and between insurers and consumers, letting market forces do their work. But this theoretical picture ignores how the USS *Health Care* has been constructed over many decades in response to Americans' values. The history of those public investments in the social good of US health care is the focus of the rest of this chapter.

Two lessons warrant emphasis. First, market efficiency and community accountability are both important. Health policies that frustrate either value should be retooled or eliminated. Second, market efficiency can be valued as an end in itself or as a means to another goal. FQHC policy is an example of valuing market efficiency as a means to community accountability. Conservatives often leap from identifying inefficiencies in US health care to concluding that market efficiency must be pursued for its own sake. A pure efficiency approach to market reform easily tolerates cutting people off from uncompensated care. Some people will miscalculate their risks and fail to purchase adequate insurance coverage. Other people will lack the resources to purchase either insurance or routine care, even with vouchers and tax credits. Yet in the face of this unmet need, Americans will not stand for shutting off access to emergency care, however inefficient it is. Over the decades, the public and philanthropic commitments invested in US health care have built up cultural attitudes of compassion and solidarity and social norms of equity and shared responsibility making pure market efficiency a nonstarter.

Public policies reflect social values and establish social priorities. DSH payments and FQHC funding answer to a vision of health care as a social good that

starts with recognizing our common vulnerability to illness, injury, and disability. Yet the commitment to community accountability cannot be one-sided
because market efficiency matters, too. On the question of how to reduce our
reliance on emergency care as a key piece of the nation's efforts at community
accountability, readers will likely judge FQHC policy as the better route to
affordable, quality care for all. Although DSH payments fund much more than
emergency care, they have facilitated the overuse of emergency departments.
FQHC funding brings primary care to people living in underserved areas, doing
a better job of balancing community accountability with market efficiency.

This judgment in favor of FQHCs informs the ACA. In addition to the $12
billion for capital investment, the Act extends market-rate Medicaid reimbursements to the growing number of FQHCs. By contrast, DSH payments start
plummeting in 2014, dropping to a quarter of prior funding levels with somewhat higher levels for the most burdened hospitals.[23] With Medicaid slated to
cover every American earning up to 133 percent of the federal poverty level and
with millions more mandated to buy subsidized insurance, emergency departments will see fewer uninsured patients, and more insured patients will seek care
in community health centers.[24] In the jargon of health policy, the ACA redirects
DSH payments toward FQHC funding, steering public resources away from
emergency departments to primary care facilities serving MUAs and MUPs. In
place of a reactive top-down effort at equity for hospitals, the Act invites a
proactive responsibility shared among newly insured patients, nonprofit stakeholders, and the American citizens whose taxes pay most of the expense. Thus
efforts at market efficiency can transpire within a commitment to community
accountability.

BUILDING THE HUB-AND-SPOKE MODEL
OF AMERICAN MEDICINE

This overview of the health care safety net teaches somewhat contradictory lessons. The world's wealthiest society has lessened the problem of uncompensated
care by building a backstop of compassion, equity, and solidarity into public
policies extending care to uninsured and poor patients. Yet even here, market-
oriented FQHC policies promise lower-cost care and improved health outcomes. For many conservatives this apparent contradiction adds up to a clear
conclusion: Americans should roll back government regulation and public insurance programs in favor of a market-driven system. American medicine could be
a nimble, entrepreneurial private system, they argue, were it not bogged down

by schizophrenic public policies of unlimited entitlements to health care and rigid price controls on providers. The failures of the safety net demonstrate, in their judgment, that the private good of health care has been derailed from its natural, rational course by public efforts to make it a social good.

This conservative line of argument echoes one of the central stories of twentieth-century American medicine. Prior to the ACA, the American Medical Association (AMA) fought every effort to implement a national health plan, public insurance program, or other comprehensive health care reform. In this narrative private physicians pursuing the best medicine and the best interests of their patients saved US health care from the path of socialized medicine, a term that has been so historically fluid as to become practically meaningless in an American context. In the 1930s President Franklin D. Roosevelt was so fearful of AMA opposition to a national health insurance plan that he left it out of his Social Security legislation. The AMA branded President Harry Truman's national health insurance bill socialized medicine, and the association applied the same label to Medicare and Medicaid in the 1960s and subsequent reform proposals, too.[25] At its core, the charge of socialized medicine appears to reject any effort to finance or structure US health care around collective public ends instead of private voluntary purposes. This public good–private good distinction presupposes that the successes of American medicine have been achieved by holding government financing and policy goals at bay.

On the contrary, US health care would be unrecognizable without its public-private partnerships. Public funding has shaped the most taken-for-granted features of twentieth-century American medicine—acute care hospitals, intensive specialization, research innovation, and technological prowess. Although Truman lost his battle for national health insurance, under his administration public investment in hospital construction and medical research exploded, inaugurating the federal government's role as a major funder, regulator, and provider (in that order) of US health care.[26]

Sociologist Paul Starr lists three phases in the "succession of objectives in medical policy" since the 1940s: expansion, equity, and cost containment.[27] Starting with expansion, the principal tool was a public-private partnership model of federal seed money for health care facility construction and federal funding of independent scientists. The 1946 Hill-Burton Act authorized federal loans and grants for building and improving community hospitals and, as amended in 1954, nursing homes. During the program's twenty-five years, $3.7 billion in federal funding enticed an "estimated $9.1 billion in local and state matching funds." As these figures are in historical dollars, a more telling statistic is that Hill-Burton funds contributed to 30 percent of hospital projects in the period.[28] This hospital build-out was matched by an outpouring of federally sponsored medical research. Up to 1945, private investments had dwarfed public expenditures. That year, pharmaceutical companies led the pack, providing $40 million in research spending, while private foundations, universities, and research institutes added $25 million. The Public Health Service made the largest federal investment in medical research, spending $3 million—an enormous sum compared to the National Institute of Health's paltry budget of $180,000. Reconstituted in 1948 as the plural National Institutes of Health (NIH), federal research funding rose to $46.3 million in 1950 and $400 million by 1960. From 1941 to 1951, the percentage of public funding in national medical research expenditures leapt from 17 percent to 42 percent.[29]

Despite embracing these funding inducements for new medical infrastructure and research, the AMA resisted federal funding of medical training as an intrusion on physician autonomy. Even so, the GI Bill subsidized the rapid growth in hospital residency programs after World War II. It provided direct funds to the veterans in the programs and indirect funds to their sponsoring hospitals, contributing to the boom in specialties and specialists in American medicine. As a result of the Hill-Burton hospital build-out and the specialized medical training it encouraged, the balance of power in the AMA shifted away from the independent practitioners who had dominated the organization, opening the way for expanded funding of graduate medical education through the new Medicare program.[30] As Starr observes, "Between 1965 and 1980, federal aid succeeded in increasing the number of medical schools from 88 to 126 and raising the number of graduates from 7,409 to 15,135."[31]

Not only did US health policy fuel expansion, but expansion of a particular sort. In the hub-and-spoke model of American medicine, community hospitals are the hub, and primary care doctors line the rim of the wheel. Radiating out along the spokes are the specialists who provide focused care and refer patients to the community hospital. Teaching hospitals serve as the training grounds for physicians and the research centers for medical innovation. Most Americans take this organizational structure for granted in seeking care, but in fact, the hub-and-spoke model faces many questions and challenges today.

Consider the abundance of specialists in the United States compared to other advanced health care systems.[32] One explanation lies in the steadily rising aid to hospitals for medical education. In the 1980s, graduate medical education (GME) funds were divided into direct medical education (DME) payments to teaching hospitals on a per-resident basis and indirect medical education (IME) payments to offset the larger share of uninsured patients that teaching hospitals serve. In 2009, Medicare contributed $9.5 billion for medical education ($3 billion for DME and $6.5 billion for IME).[33] Forty-one states added $3.8 billion in Medicaid GME funds.[34] States injected another $5 billion through medical school appropriations. This public funding of $18.3 billion for medical schools and residency programs outpaced by six to one the $2.9 billion in tuition and fees that medical students paid for their education that year.[35]

This extraordinarily high level of public subsidies for medical education puts physicians' complaints about the cost of their training in a different light. Direct comparisons between public subsidies and private tuition are admittedly difficult because medical school lasts four years while residency programs vary in length. Furthermore, IME payments support hospitals not residents, and even DME payments mostly flow to hospitals rather than to underpaid residents. Factoring in these caveats, a cautious estimate suggests public subsidies of more than two to one for the average physician's training.

Incurring student loans of several hundred thousand dollars is a very heavy burden. It is understandable, therefore, that some physicians develop an acute sense of individual ownership over their medical training and feel entitled to the rich salaries commanded by specialists who perform remunerative procedures. This attitude presupposes that medical education is a private good, one that is earned by people who have paid their dues in time and money. To this way of thinking, physicians have made personal and financial sacrifices for some time period, so they have fully paid for their medical knowledge. Now they should be free to charge patients a price set by the same market mechanisms that dictate the price of a medical education.

Protestant ethicist William F. May challenges the notion of medical education as a private good and its accompanying attitudes. He argues that physicians enter into a covenant in their training that links them to past generations of pioneering physicians and sacrificing patients whose trial-and-error experiments yielded the gifts of medical knowledge. As with all covenants, May writes, the originating gifts "require a fidelity that exceeds any specification."[36] In the case of medical training, the physician's proper response is the professional obligation to make return sacrifices exceeding monetary payment alone. Also demanded is a fidelity to excellence in one's medical practice and to the generous spirit of the original patients who sacrificed for the health of unknown others.

Public subsidies for medical education do not have the same moral weight as the gifts that May describes. They are more social contract than covenantal gift. Public support for medical training is an investment with social returns. Were physicians-in-training expected to pay the full cost of their education, US health care would suffer from a critical shortage of physicians. Moreover, educating doctors, nurses, and other health professionals requires universities staffed by scientists conducting cutting-edge research and by health professionals practiced in highly technical skills. The achievements of academic medicine explain why Americans have not only invested heavily in teaching hospitals and university research but also granted physicians a social monopoly through board certification and state laws. Americans have maintained their generous support of graduate medical education because they recognize its social value. Indeed, medical education demonstrates how pervasively this foundational aspect of US health care has been organized as a social good.[37]

Public support for medical research tells a similar story. Private industry still invests the most in medical research, spending $58.6 billion in 2007 compared to $38 billion spent by federal, state, and local governments.[38] But government is the principal funder of basic research into the causes of disease. Industry support steps up as a drug comes to market, increasing at each stage from drug discovery to design to manufacturing to final approval when profitable sales begin. In fact, industry-sponsored research has shifted funding from pharmaceuticals to medical devices, where the larger profit margins now lie. The remaining pharmaceutical research focuses so much on modifying existing molecular entities instead of creating new classes of drugs that in 2001, the NIH established the National Center for Advancing Translational Sciences, a venture that journalist Gardiner Harris has described as "akin to that of a home seller who spruces up properties to attract buyers in a down market. In this case the center will do as much research as it needs to do so that it can attract drug company investment."[39] While comprising only a small portion of total medical research dollars, philanthropic support by foundations and individual donors ($4.3 billion in 2007) is also directed toward basic research and design of new molecules and therapies, much more so than the risk-averse strategies of today's pharmaceutical giants.[40]

Although private industry continues to exceed government and philanthropic spending, their respective research priorities reflect the competing pulls of market efficiency and community accountability. Private industry's research is geared toward blockbuster medicines that patients take for an extended period of time or throughout their lives. Biotechnology firms produce niche medicines for small markets where there are few competitors and high prices. By comparison, mass-produced, low-cost drugs are economically inefficient in terms of their financial payback. For example, annual flu vaccinations, taken once for only one season, have broad public health benefits and tremendous social value. Without federal support, however, they will be underproduced by companies seeking to recoup their investments over the long term. In total, US health care would lose 38 percent of its research investment without government funding. More importantly, this loss would curtail the development of therapies with the widest benefits for most Americans' health.[41]

Government support of medical infrastructure, training, and research illustrates how thoroughly US health care has been organized as a social good. Clearly, public financing and policy goals have by no means been restricted to safety-net programs. The hub-and-spoke model was built in the image of legislated social priorities, starting with the financial incentives that made hospitals the hubs of a highly specialized medical workforce that rewards the provision of acute care and the search for miracle cures. Hospitals remain the hubs through which medical training and research dollars flow with concentrated force. Americans have shared in the cost of these efforts because of the widespread benefits of medical innovation and excellence. Expanding the research, training, and delivery infrastructure exceeded the capacity of private organizations and required the extensive social investment that defines all social goods.

MEDICARE AND MEDICAID: PUBLIC INSURANCE AND COST CONTROL

Turning to the second and third phases of US health policy—equity and cost control—the Medicare and Medicaid programs take center stage. Having built US health care together, Americans moved to share it and then struggled to control its rising costs. A comparison of the two programs reveals Americans' ambivalence about committing fully to health care solidarity. It also demonstrates the high cost of a partial solidarity that pursues equity through massive social investments in expanded capacity with little social coordination on behalf of the social priorities of wellness, prevention, and cost-effective care.

The names of Medicare and Medicaid reflect the different attitudes that Americans bring to them. Medicare, the federal program for elderly and disabled Americans, enjoys the strong legitimacy of a program into which all working Americans contribute payroll taxes and from which nearly all seniors benefit. These two factors—the payroll tax for the hospital portion of Medicare and the near universality of benefits—make Medicare a social insurance program, a shared insurance system in which every contributor becomes a beneficiary. Thus the "care" of Medicare is viewed as equity by addition. Including elderly and disabled people in US health care is achieved by *adding* a funding stream to cover *additional* recipients who enjoy the same benefits as all other seniors. Once again, however, we find a discrepancy between public attitudes and the structural realities of US health care. Medicare also achieves equity through redistribution, the complaint directed against Medicaid. Today's seniors enjoy an average payout rate of four to one compared to the "lifetime value" of their payroll taxes into the system.[42]

Medicaid is viewed as redistributive aid, not intergenerational care. This aid has flowed not only to eligible low-income children, pregnant women, nursing home residents, and disabled Americans but also to those states with proportionately more low-income residents.[43] Medicaid's lack of a dedicated payroll tax and its lack of universality explain the program's low reimbursement levels. Many Americans feel limited solidarity with Medicaid beneficiaries, so fewer efforts are made to ensure that all Americans would be willing to live with the reality of Medicaid health care. Yet this attitude of distant charity clashes with the fact that Medicaid covered 62 million Americans in 2012—nearly 20 percent of the total population.[44] Beginning in 2014, the ACA is designed to transform Medicaid from a social welfare program for Americans who cannot work due to age, disability, or maternal obligations into a foundational guarantee for Americans in families earning up to 133 percent of the federal poverty level. The ACA acknowledges that many working poor cannot afford health insurance. Although Medicaid remains equity by redistribution, its more negative associations may dissipate with its cultural transformation from social welfare to social guarantee.[45]

The push for equity in US health care is inseparable from the pull of cost control. One reason is that President Lyndon Johnson agreed to generous Medicare reimbursements in an effort to win the AMA's support for the proposed law. As a result, hospitals were initially paid on a "cost-plus" basis, and physicians retained their fee-for-service payments. Thus Medicare did not alter the patient-dollar-service linkage in US health care. It simply primed the pump by increasing payments into the hub-and-spoke system.

Health economist Amy Finkelstein has calculated the catalytic jolt that Medicare gave to this system of technology-driven, specialized acute care. Examining Medicare's first decade, from 1965 to 1975, she finds surprisingly different effects on coverage rates and health outcomes. In its first year Medicare increased hospital insurance rates for elderly Americans from an average of 25 percent across the country to nearly 100 percent.[46] Seniors gained financial security as out-of-pocket costs tumbled for patients with the highest medical expenses. By contrast, the data on mortality rates show no improvement. Medicare had no discernible effect on seniors' mortality rate during its first decade because, prior to 1965, elderly Americans with legal access to health care were able to receive life-saving services that were paid for by their own out-of-pocket spending or hospital insurance or that were donated by hospitals as charity care.[47] At least initially, Medicare afforded seniors financial security, but not improved mortality rates.

Medicare's other immediate effect was to increase the overall cost of US health care. The influx of Medicare funds changed health care not simply by degree but in kind. Medicare payments prompted providers to make systemic changes, notably in the acquisition of advanced technology by hospitals. Finkelstein's data corrects previous estimates based on the famous Rand Corporation's Health Insurance Experiment, which analyzed how individuals react to changes in their insurance coverage and copays. By aggregating individual decisions about health care usage, the Rand researchers concluded that Medicare's introduction increased US health care costs by 5.6 percent. Finkelstein's data shows that the jump was at least 23 percent during Medicare's first five years. How can we make sense of this discrepancy? The answer is that aggregating individual decisions is an insufficient model. The Rand methodology cannot account for the systemic factors emphasized by Finkelstein, including the "dynamic feedback loop" generated by Medicare's guaranteed funding of such expensive and technology-intensive services as cardiac care. As Finkelstein notes, the "arrival rate" of advanced technology accelerated not only for seniors but also for patients across the board.[48]

The Rand experiment investigated such micro-level changes as how many more services individuals purchase when they gain insurance coverage and how much they cut back when their copays rise. This information is useful as far as it goes. When a social choice is made to invest in health coverage for a whole class of people, however, the entire system also changes. As a result of Medicare's new taxes and entitlements, Americans came to share even more in one another's health risks and health care costs. Once again we have evidence of how broadly US health care had become a social good.

Today we face a situation in which public attitudes and assumptions do not cohere with the structural realities and shared values of US health care. Americans are in the habit of eyeing other people's health care entitlements suspiciously without recognizing how the public funds that flow to some people's care also support the broader health care infrastructure, knowledge base, and professional skills that serve the many. Similarly, when providers complain about their low Medicare and Medicaid reimbursements, they ignore the larger budget picture. The fixed costs of technology-dependent hospitals (and increasingly outpatient services) demand the guaranteed funding of Medicare and Medicaid. In 2010, public payers covered $964 billion of Americans' health care spending compared to the $829 billion paid by private insurers and the $294 billion paid by consumers out-of-pocket. Medicare ($500 billion) and Medicaid

($374 billion) have improved access for elderly, disabled, and poor Americans.[49] They have subsidized the health care safety net through DSH and FQHC payments and physician training through GME grants. Their payments for hospital and medical services have enlarged the hospital sector in particular and increased the growth of US health care in general.

Finkelstein's Medicare data teach another important lesson. Even if Medicare's primary goal was equity for seniors, it transpired within the context of the expansionist policies that preceded it. If we stop to rank the shared values served by US health policy, we find that innovation, excellence, and equity have run far ahead of efficiency and stewardship. Given the tenuous safety-net commitments to Medicaid recipients and to emergency care for uninsured patients, compassion and solidarity stand somewhere in the middle. The social good of US health care must be evaluated in light of all of the shared values meant to be served by public funding and the delivery structures it supports. Examining US health care through this wide-angle lens, we see that it is an incomplete social good that needs much better social coordination alongside the many social investments that Americans have made.

Public efforts to coordinate US health care date to the 1980s when the third goal of US health policy—cost containment—became a leading concern. At that time Medicare's retrospective cost-plus payments to hospitals were replaced by a prospective payment system that classified thousands of medical conditions into diagnosis-related groups, each with a flat fee. Medicare also added a new payment scale for physicians. These reimbursement mechanisms shifted payments away from individual patient care to average patient care. Instead of covering all of the services ordered for an individual patient, payments were fixed at expected services for an average patient with a certain diagnosis. As a result, Medicare's payments fell below private insurers' reimbursements and slowed the growth of public spending. Thus health economist Uwe Reinhardt could conclude in 1996 that government is not "the chief culprit in the rising cost of health care." Instead "private employers actually have been the chief cost drivers in the American health system."[50]

How does Reinhardt's claim square with Finkelstein's finding of large cost increases in Medicare's first decade? Recall the image of the USS *Health Care*. Public payers established the funding platform on which US health care built up the ship and its armamentarium of treatment options. The social investment in public insurance, along with the earlier subsidies for medical infrastructure, research, and training, greatly expanded the care options for individual patients and increased the expense of this intensive care. Private insurers and the employers and workers who pay insurance premiums have also been willing participants in this unchecked growth. By paying higher reimbursements, private insurers seem to be playing fairly, unlike the government, by compensating providers for their costs plus a bit more. Looking at the growth patterns in capital spending and service lines in US health care, however, providers are always seeking to attract privately insured patients, luring them with the latest technology, the newest treatments, and the fanciest facilities. With private insurers more willing to pay the extra costs of this high-end care, they are effectively the high-test fuel that keeps the USS *Health Care* churning forward at faster and faster speeds.

This chapter has described the many ways that US health care has been organized as a social good. Through the vehicle of health policy, Americans have invested in medical research, training, and infrastructure, supported public insurance programs for the elderly, the disabled, and the poor, and mandated uncompensated care. Once we consider the tax subsidies for employer-sponsored private insurance (see chapter 1), it is clear that the health policy push for shared funding of quality health care has been remarkably expansive. It has not been systematically coordinated, however. To return to this chapter's epigraph, speaking the language of common good is "nonsensical" in a political system that aspires to "enlightened self-interest." But an "our" commitment to pay for a health care system that operates with a "my" mentality remains viable only as long as unchecked funding allows expansion to drive the ship and equity to be meted out to a greater (Medicare) or lesser degree (Medicaid and uncompensated care). In developing US health care, Americans have devoted much greater attention to social investments in high-powered medicine and social recognition of unmet need than they have to social priorities of wellness, prevention, and cost-effective care. Today this third leg of the stool—cost containment—is shorter and less developed than the other two, leaving US health care teetering on the verge of unsustainability.

THE SOCIAL IMPLICATIONS OF THE INDIVIDUAL MANDATE

The Affordable Care Act nudges US health care toward a more coherent social good. Despite being called an individual mandate, the law's requirement that most Americans obtain health coverage for themselves and their families reflects two social realities. First, in response to shared vulnerability to disease and disability, Americans have made compassion and solidarity backstop values of US health policy. Uninsured patients have access to care, however limited and inconvenient. Second, Americans have pooled enormous resources in building

US health care and maintaining an array of remarkable health care options. The individual mandate conjoins these two social realities. Because Americans have access to care that would bankrupt all but the few, everyone is obliged to obtain health coverage to expand the funding base and extend the sharing of health care costs. This balancing act plays throughout the ACA. To ensure coverage for the poorest Americans, Medicaid expands. To help moderate-income Americans afford mandated coverage, new public subsidies defray the cost of premiums, deductibles, and copays. To curb excessive insurance premiums, rules limit insurers' ability to rate health policies according to individual risk. Taken together, such changes make the payment system for US health care even more of a shared endeavor.

By contrast, market reformers champion the "my" mentality of the patient-dollar-service payment system that most Americans assume already funds US health care. The idea behind market reform is simple. US health care should reflect what individual Americans value. Although simple in theory, market reform is revolutionary in policy, rejecting the shared values built into the social good of US health care and replacing them with the short-term preferences of those consumers with the financial resources to enter the health care market. Under this approach, expansion would be checked by consumer choice and redirected toward efficient innovation at a better price. The concept of equity would narrow, becoming in practice equal benefits for equal payments into the system.

The philosophical gap between the visions of health care as a private choice and health care as a social good was on display during oral arguments before the US Supreme Court in March 2012. Arguing in favor of the ACA, Solicitor General Donald Verrilli appealed to the social norm of providing uncompensated care and to the social structures of managing health risks cooperatively. The court's conservative justices kept their focus on individuals' choices and risks in the insurance market.

The individual mandate raises the important constitutional question, Can the federal government mandate the purchase of health insurance through its powers to regulate interstate commerce? But during oral arguments, two other questions emerged as more fundamental: Does the social norm of providing uncompensated care have any binding effect on individuals' decisions about whether or not to have health insurance? Do the existing social structures for managing health risks through private and public insurance, on the one hand, and through public spending on medical research, training, and infrastructure, on the other hand, in any way curtail individual liberty in assessing one's own health risks?

On the question of publicly sanctioned social norms, Justice Antonin Scalia argued that the Tenth Amendment's limits on federal power require leaving "the people . . . to decide whether they want to buy insurance or not." Describing young and healthy people without insurance, he added, "These people are not stupid. They're going to buy insurance later. They're young and need the money now."[51] For Scalia, when individuals take a calculated risk in choosing not to purchase insurance, they do not enter the insurance market. Therefore, federal law has no authority over their "inactivity" because no commerce has occurred. Countering this argument, Verrilli set individual health insurance decisions in the context of public policies guaranteeing access to emergency care. Americans who choose not to purchase insurance know they are guaranteed care in emergency departments. In Verrilli's words, "You're going into [the health care] market without the ability to pay, [but] you're getting the health care service anyway as a result of the social norms . . . to which we've obligated ourselves so that people can get health care." Getting to the crux of disagreement, Scalia retorted, "Well, don't obligate yourself to that!"[52] In Scalia's thinking, an individual's decision not to purchase a health insurance policy is separable from any social values enshrined in federal laws guaranteeing emergency care. Individual preferences stand free and clear of the social values of solidarity and compassion, regardless of their having been legislated through democratic processes and woven into the fabric of the health care system.

On the question of existing social structures for managing health risk, Justice Anthony Kennedy argued that individuals are free to decide their own risks, and the government cannot intrude paternalistically on individuals' judgments. With the individual mandate, he claimed, "the government is saying that the Federal Government has a duty to tell the individual citizen that it must act. . . . In the law of torts, our tradition, our law has been that you don't have the duty to rescue someone if that person is in danger."[53] Kennedy sees the individual mandate in terms of rescue—that the government is rescuing people from potential harm to themselves by requiring them to obtain insurance rather than simply enticing their purchase with new public subsidies. Individuals should be at liberty, Kennedy implies, to buy a policy or not buy a policy at their own personal and financial risk.

In US health care, however, individual risk and harm are hard to separate from social risk and harm. As Justice Sonia Sotomayor observed, "If you use health services, you have to pay with insurance, because only health insurance will guarantee that whatever need for health care that you have will be paid for, because virtually no one, perhaps with the exception of 1 percent of the population, can afford the massive cost if the unexpected happens."[54] Beginning with the group policies of employer-sponsored insurance, these private health insurance policies are de facto agreements to rescue one another when health risk turns into expensive health need. Public insurance extends this commitment to mutual rescue even further. The guaranteed provision of uncompensated care through all of the safety-net funding detailed above secures a semblance of rescue for the uninsured, too. Finally, public investments in medical training, research, and infrastructure help ensure that excellent care is at the ready when health crises strike. Once health care has been structured in this way as a social good, it is no longer simply a matter of individual risk and harm. The individual risk of unbearable expense is borne as a social risk. When individuals lack adequate insurance, "my" individual harm becomes "our" social harm.

Today the organization of US health care is shaped by the social norm of guaranteeing uncompensated care and by the social structures of sharing in and responding to one another's health risks and health care costs. As market reformers look to dismantle the social good of US health care, they must answer two sets of questions. First, for Americans who are priced out of the health insurance market or who choose not to enter it, what provision, if any, should be made for their care? Most importantly, will the social norm of guaranteeing uncompensated care be preserved or abandoned? Second, if uninsured Americans are not to be cut adrift from the USS *Health Care*, then who will pay the cost of the care they cannot afford? Assuming that taxpayers and privately insured people will continue to bear the costs of uncovered individuals' risk, how will the public be protected against bearing even higher costs if, as is likely, the rolls of the uninsured rise with the onset of market reform?

These two challenges clarify the differences between social goods and other necessities. One difference lies in the sheer cost of social goods and the need to pool resources to pay for them. Food stamps and housing assistance help individuals pay for the necessities of food and shelter, but the burden of paying for catastrophic health care, like the cost of building one's own system of fire protection, clean water, or universal education, exceeds individuals' capacity. The other, more important difference lies in the fact that investing in social goods together is warranted because the benefits are so widespread as to be social, not individual. When people lack food and shelter, the individual harm is grave, but the social harm generally is not. With social goods, the concern is not only the individual harm but also the social harms that follow directly in its wake. With health care, they include the public health effects of contagion as well as the economic costs of the nation's policy commitments to pay for uncompensated care.

It is difficult to speak the language of the social good of "our" health care not only in Congress and the marketplace but also in the Supreme Court. Nevertheless, Americans have made longstanding policy commitments to the values of care and respect, innovation and fairness, and compassion and solidarity in building and steering the USS *Health Care* through decades of public policy. Recognizing that US health care is a social good does not mean, however, that the ways it serves the members of this society are always *good*. The term describes instead how much health care has been organized as a community resource through shared funding and shared management of risk. US health care's most obvious deficiency has been the inability to control costs or serve the social priorities of wellness, prevention, and cost-effectiveness.

Part 2 of the book moves into the domain of religious health care nonprofits whose philanthropic efforts are another source of shared values in US health care. I argue that taking stock of this fuller spectrum of shared values confirms the wisdom of health care reform that makes US health care a more fully coherent social good.

NOTES

1. Barr, *Introduction to US Health Policy*, 35.
2. Ibid., 36–37.
3. Mackey, "The Whole Foods Alternative to ObamaCare," *Wall Street Journal* Aug. 11, 2009; quoted in Barr, *Introduction*, 14.
4. Martin et al., "Growth in US Health Spending Remained Slow in 2010," 212.
5. In an interesting use of the term social good, David Stockman, President Ronald Reagan's budget director, argued that health care is an economic good, lamenting that it is instead viewed "as sort of a spiritual, collective, or social good. As a consequence it is treated, regulated, and managed by society in a unique way that departs from the way in which markets normally handle other economic goods" (quoted in Iglehart, "Health Care USA").
6. Zoloth, *Health Care and the Ethics of Encounter*, 50.
7. Care for chronic illnesses is estimated to absorb 75 percent of US health care expenditures (Centers for Disease Control, "Chronic Diseases," 2).
8. Cunningham, "Nonurgent Use of Emergency Departments," 4–5, 11.
9. Finkelstein, "The Aggregate Effects of Health Insurance," 4.
10. Finkelstein and McKnight, "What Did Medicare Do (And Was It Worth It)?" 3.
11. In 2012, 16 percent of covered workers were enrolled in a health maintenance organization, down from a high of 31 percent in 1996 (Kaiser Family Foundation, "Exhibit 5.1," *Employer Health Benefits 2012*).
12. Hadley et al. ("Covering the Uninsured in 2008," w403) estimate that in 2008 hospitals provided $35 billion in uncompensated care and received $28.7 billion in direct (e.g., DSH payments) and indirect (e.g., IME funds) subsidies.

13. According to Barr, "Physicians in many areas of the country receive only 30 to 40 percent of their usual charge for taking care of a Medicaid patient. As a result of these payment policies, in 2006 only 52 percent of physicians were willing to accept new patients on Medicaid" (*Introduction*, 174). Using costs instead of charges brings Medicaid reimbursements much closer to Medicare and commercial insurance; see American Hospital Association, "Aggregate Hospital Payment-to-Cost Ratios."

14. Martin et al., "Growth in US Health Spending," 213.

15. McKethan et al., "Reforming the Medicaid Disproportionate-Share Hospital Program," w927–28.

16. Kaiser Family Foundation, "Federal Medicaid Disproportionate Share (DSH) Allotments"; and Nguyen and Sheingold, "Indirect Medical Education," E2.

17. Health Resources and Service Administration, US Department of Health and Human Services, "Health Center Data." http://bphc.hrsa.gov/uds/view.aspx?year= 2010 (accessed Apr. 20, 2012).

18. According to an industry group, the National Association of Community Health Centers ("Community Health Centers"), FQHCs are reimbursed only 81 percent of their cost per patient.

19. Kaiser Family Foundation, "United States: Federally Qualified Health Centers, 2010 Data."

20. Kaiser Health News, "National Health Service Corp. Nearly Triples in Size, According to HHS," Oct. 14, 2011.

21. Iglehart, "Health Centers Fill Critical Gap," 343–45.

22. Beauchamp makes a similar distinction between a "consumer or 'me' psychology" and a "communal or 'we' psychology" in arguing for a national health plan (*Health Care Reform*, 97).

23. Nguyen and Sheingold, "Indirect Medical Education," E14–E15.

24. The US Supreme Court's ruling in *NFIB v. Sebelius* allowed states to opt out without penalty from the ACA's Medicaid expansion. The Congressional Budget Office projects that instead of 33 million more Americans having new coverage (by about 2020), that number will drop to 29 or 30 million ("Estimates for the Insurance Coverage Provisions," 13).

25. Hoffman, *National Health Insurance*. Barr notes that in 1932 the AMA labeled the first pre-paid health maintenance organizations unethical "medical Soviets" (*Introduction*, 105). Rothman takes a more positive view, stressing the "entrepreneurial" and "voluntary" ethos of American medicine in explaining the repeated failures of national health care reform ("Century of Failure," 278–82).

26. Starr, *The Social Transformation of American Medicine*, 276–81.

27. Ibid., 338.

28. Ibid., 348, 350.

29. Ibid., 342–43, 347.

30. Rich et al., "Medicare Financing of Graduate Medical Education," 284.

31. Starr, *Social Transformation*, 421.

32. As Barr notes, "The greater the number of physicians, the greater has been the amount of care and the number of procedures. Instead of reducing the price of care, the rising number of specialist physicians has contributed to the increasing cost of care" (*Introduction*, 85).

33. Medicare Payment Advisory Commission, *Aligning Incentives in Medicare*, 103.

34. Henderson, *Medicaid Direct and Indirect Graduate Medical Education Payments*, 6.

35. Association of American Medical Colleges, "Table 6."

36. May, "Code, Covenant, Contract, or Philanthropy," 30–31.

37. Callahan predicts a loss of public funding for medical education and research under market reform ("Medicine and the Market," 233).

38. Dorsey et al., "Funding of US Biomedical Research," 139.

39. Harris, "Federal Research Center Will Help Develop Medicines."

40. Moses and Martin, "Biomedical Research and Health Advances," 567–68.

41. Federal, state, and local governments spent another $69 billion in 2007 on such public health programs as "epidemiological surveillance, inoculations, immunization/vaccine services, disease prevention programs, the operation of public health laboratories" (US Census Bureau, "Table 135").

42. Steuerle and Rennane, "Social Security and Medicare Taxes and Benefits over a Lifetime," 2–3.

43. Prior to the ACA, poorer states received as high as a 74 percent federal match on Medicaid spending compared to an average match of 57 percent.

44. Kaiser Commission on Medicaid and the Uninsured, "Five Key Questions about Medicaid," 2.

45. In Chief Justice Roberts's majority ruling, "Under the Affordable Care Act . . . , [Medicaid] is no longer a program to care for the neediest among us, but rather an element of a comprehensive national health plan to provide universal health insurance coverage." See *NFIB v. Sebelius*, 53–54. The decision by many states not to expand Medicaid hinders this social guarantee for the poorest Americans.

46. Finkelstein, "Aggregate Effects," 4.

47. Finkelstein and McKnight, "What Did Medicare Do," 1–2.

48. Finkelstein, "Aggregate Effects," 25–26, 30–31. Ginzberg confirms that Medicare's cost-plus reimbursements allowed suburban hospitals to update into good tertiary facilities ("Health-Care Policy in the United States in the 20th Century," 71). Medical technology still accounts "for an estimated 38 percent to more than 65 percent of spending increases" (Robert Wood Johnson Foundation, "What Are the Biggest Drivers of Cost in US Health Care?").

49. Martin et al., "Growth in US Health Spending," 211.

50. Reinhardt, "Employer-Based Health Insurance," 332–35, 337.

51. Oral argument, *Department of Health and Human Services v. Florida*, 29, 35.

52. Ibid., 20.

53. Ibid., 31.

54. Ibid., 21–22.

Part Two

Religious Values in Health Policy, Markets, and Politics

Chapter 4

Modeling Community Benefits

SOCIAL CONTRACT, COMMON GOOD, COVENANT

We don't want to get to the end of our fiscal year, and say, "Oh my God, what did we do for community benefit? Did you do anything? Okay, did you do anything? We've got to get these numbers up." Before June 30, you should be planning for next year. What have we learned? What is our community coalition saying? What are the meanings? We're always going to take care of the uninsured and the underinsured. But what about the big picture? For the CEO, the first and last concern is the number sign. That's what your newspaper picks up, and that's what the hospital down the street looks at. It's the competitive capitalist environment, so we don't want to be naive, but [community benefit] has to be put in a different kind of lane for us.

Director of advocacy, nationwide Catholic hospital system

PART I OF THIS BOOK reviewed the three moral languages of US health care. None of them accounts for how much US health care is organized as a social good. Chapter 3 described Americans' social investments in innovation, excellence, compassion, and equity through many decades of public policy and public funding. Other shared values have entered US health care through the philanthropic commitments of nonprofit health care organizations. As noted by Lester Salamon, American nonprofit organizations have frequently been "partners in public service" with government.[1] One foundation of this partnership is the tax-exempt status granted to charitable 501(c)(3) organizations by federal, state, and local governments, an arrangement that can be viewed as a social contract. In exchange for serving public charitable purposes, private nonprofits are excused from the public obligation of paying taxes. Yet this simple picture of a social contract raises many questions. In the case of US health care, the most important one has been whether nonprofit providers are making a big enough difference in helping to meet the nation's shared responsibilities of caring for uninsured and underinsured patients.

In this chapter I take that question as the occasion for delving into the moral dialogues about mission and values inside religiously affiliated health care organizations. The epigraph to this chapter recounts the leadership discussions at one of the largest Catholic hospital systems in the country. The advocacy official was describing how her office approached the Internal Revenue Service's requirement that tax-exempt hospitals provide "community benefits." The meaning of this phrase has been hotly contested since the IRS promulgated the community benefit standard in 1969. In recent decades a wide array of critics, from Sen. Charles Grassley (R-IA) on the right to the Service Employees International Union on the left, have charged nonprofit hospitals with failing to provide enough uncompensated care to warrant their favorable tax status.

Looking at the data, a 2006 review of empirical studies found it difficult to conclude definitively that nonprofit and for-profit "ownership 'matters' in health care." Nevertheless, there is "consistent evidence" that nonprofit hospitals are "more oriented toward the local community and more likely to provide specific services that benefit the community." Nonprofit hospitals also "remain consistently more accessible to indigent and other unprofitable clients," and they are "less likely [to have] high markups on their charges for services."[2] These national trends vary depending on local health care markets. Moreover, being community oriented is not the same as dedicating the full value of one's tax exemptions to uncompensated care, which is what critics of nonprofit hospitals have been urging.[3] Public scrutiny has focused most intensely on nonprofit providers with a religious mission.

The effects of this scrutiny can be heard in the advocacy official's account of the frantic search for more quantifiable community benefits in past fiscal years. From the very top of her organization on down, the drive was for a big-dollar figure of community benefits to impress the media and to surpass the competitor down the street, especially if that competitor was a for-profit hospital required to pay taxes. This anecdote highlights the tension between external measures of a nonprofit's charitable purpose and the internal priorities of an organization serving its mission and values. In the advocacy director's words, "It's the competitive capitalist environment, so we don't want to be naive, but it has to be put in a different kind of lane for us." This image captures how religious providers have to travel in the health care market, heeding the same number signs, but trying to steer their own course. The question is whether the expressway of US health care allows for the community benefits that religious providers aspire to, or whether they are propelled along with every other hospital in the race after capital-intensive, high-priced specialty care to attract privately insured patients.

The pressures come not only from the health care marketplace. Pressure has intensified on the policy side, too, in the form of legal benchmarks that would require nonprofit hospitals to devote a minimum percentage of their annual revenues or operating costs to uncompensated care. These charity care mandates have been implemented in several states and debated at the federal level. In light of the argument in chapter 3 that US health is an incomplete social good, a charity care mandate might seem like a logical and necessary extension of the public value of equity in US health care. Mandating a fixed percentage of uncompensated care for all nonprofit hospitals would ease the burden on safety-net hospitals by steering more dollars toward uncompensated care for uninsured and underinsured patients. I argue in this chapter, however, that a charity care mandate confuses the proper role of nonprofit organizations in US health care.

The shared responsibilities for health care divide into two categories: social responsibility and social responsiveness. Social responsibility has a societal reach that is comprehensive in scope and basic in obligation. To be socially responsible in health care means to structure an entire system so that all eligible people have access to services. Social responsiveness is narrower in scope and contingent in its obligations. To be socially responsive means to respond to the health needs of local communities and to partner with other organizations to maintain healthy communities. A charity care mandate equates nonprofit tax exemptions with uncompensated care obligations. While uncompensated care should be expected, especially of religious nonprofits, equating religious mission with charity care is as shortsighted as the denominational arguments for a right to health care reviewed in chapter 2. What gets lost in a debate focused on charity care is the broader social visions of common good and covenant that direct religiously committed people into action in meeting their shared responsibilities for healing.

ARTICULATING RELIGIOUS
VALUES IN HEALTH CARE

Before turning to the national debate about the community-benefit standard, a word about my research interviews is in order. My interview study is qualitative, not quantitative. I sought to listen in on the internal conversations about mission and values in Catholic and Jewish health care systems. I focused on my interviewees' moral aspirations as they invoked their core values to explain their organization's efforts to address the practical realities of US health care. I am not offering evidence that religious providers surpass secular nonprofits or for-profit competitors in quality, affordability, or accessibility of health care. Neither do I have the organizational data to confirm or dispute interviewees' claims to distinctive service in meeting their mission and values.

Nevertheless, I learned one telling measure of values in an organization. Values make a difference only to the extent that they are implemented throughout an organization's structures. During my study, I heard many stories of success (and few stories of failure) of organizations living out their mission and values. The anecdotal quality of the stories gave them an after-the-fact quality, however, that often seemed to be designed to elicit my agreement that the organization was performing admirably. But values are not the morals of stories, nor can they only be aspirational. Values must be made explicit time and again through ongoing debate within an organization, and they must be made concrete by building delivery structures that articulate the values anew. By articulate I do not mean simply speaking the values. I use the term in the sense of an articulated limb that has a specific structure related to its operations and purposes. This structure enables certain movements but not others, and its range of motion comes with limits, some of which are inherent in the structure itself and some of which arise from external forces and constraints. Critics of religious hospitals argue that these hospitals take in too much money as margin at the expense their mission. Critics decry their levels of uncompensated care as uncharitable. But these criticisms are also made after the fact. They engage in a numbers game that asks where annual revenues and costs end up instead of exploring whether religious values are concretely expressed in nonprofit structures.

Bioethicist Nancy Neveloff Dubler underscores the importance of organizational ethics to bioethics today. In her words, an "ethics of medicine that focused on the individual ethical obligations of the physician has been supplemented or supplanted by new formulations that identify the institution as the locus for moral obligation."[4] Building on this suggestion, I take the organizational structures of religious health care nonprofits as a focus of ethical inquiry and moral action. This focus fits the idea of mission integration in religious health care—that is, moving beyond simple appeals to mission and values as guiding ideals to actually working them out through discussion and implementation across an organization. This focus on structure puts the standard of judgment in the right place. We should hold nonprofit providers accountable for how well their structures of delivering care serve public charitable purposes. But we should first ensure that our assessment is informed by how the organizations themselves define their charitable purposes in light of their values.

Comparing the public debate over the community benefit standard with the conversations occurring inside religious health care organizations, we find three distinct ways to describe the public responsibility of nonprofit hospitals: as a social contract, common good, and covenant. The social contract model of community benefits is presupposed by the critics of nonprofit hospitals. In their view, nonprofit hospitals' tax exemptions are a gift from the public treasury for which a return gift of public service is due. In other words, community benefits are owed in return for lost tax revenues that the public otherwise could use to cover uninsured and underinsured patients. According to advocates of this moral framework, nonprofit hospitals are not meeting their contracted levels of charity care. In Catholic organizations leaders discuss community benefits in terms of common good. Although charity care is an essential community benefit, the real aim of these providers is to transform health care delivery structures by identifying and responding to the needs of poor and vulnerable patients, often in partnership with other organizations. In Jewish hospitals the language of covenant is a more appropriate model of community benefits. These organizations give priority to the core obligations of providing excellent medical care and serving those communities closest to their founding purposes. These more delimited covenantal obligations challenge the unbounded scope of the Catholic common good model. The argument in this chapter is framed by the two models that have dominated the public debate: the quid pro quo of a social contract and the Catholic aspiration to common good.

A recent policy development indicates how the articulation of religious values can shape US health care more generally. At the urging of hospital critics, in 2008 the IRS introduced a Schedule H reporting form for nonprofit hospitals as part of its revised Form 990, which nonprofit organizations use to report their yearly financial activities. Remarkable about Schedule H from a policy perspective is that it was modeled on the community benefits reporting guidelines developed by the Catholic Health Association (CHA) for its member hospital systems. Now the IRS may have simply decided that CHA, aided by VHA, Inc., had developed state-of-the-art accounting practices for the range of community benefits allowed under the 1969 ruling. Written into CHA's definitions, however, are moral judgments about the nature of charity care and the priority of care for poor and vulnerable patients in the ethical hierarchy of what counts as community benefits.

Specifically, Schedule H elevated two categories of community benefit above all others. At the top of the list are (1) nonprofit hospitals' losses on free and discounted care and (2) their losses on means-tested government programs, such

as Medicaid. Other community benefits, including community health improvement services, sponsored research, and health-professional education, have a
secondary billing on Schedule H. Removed from community benefits accounts
were hospitals' losses on Medicare under-reimbursements and bad debts for
patient care.[5]

The significance of these changes can be illustrated by a 2005 survey con-
ducted by the IRS. Using their own assorted definitions of community benefits,
487 nonprofit hospital respondents reported $9.3 billion in community benefits
in 2005, which broke down as follows:

> 56 percent ($5.2 billion) in uncompensated care
> 23 percent ($2.1 billion) in medical education and training
> 15 percent ($1.4 billion) in research
> 6 percent ($0.6 billion) in community programs[6]

Were we to apply current IRS reporting categories to the survey results, the
worth of the community benefits would be less. The hospitals' losses on Medicare and bad debts would be subtracted, as would any community programs—
such as medical screenings, health fairs, newsletters, support groups, and cash
and in-kind donations—that did not meet an "identifiable community need."[7]
Thus as nonprofit hospitals have adjusted to the new landscape of Schedule H,
they have come under the influence of Catholic values on community benefits
policy. Because almost three-fifths of community hospitals in the United States
are nonprofit (compared to 20 percent that are for-profit and 22 percent
government-owned), this religious influence on US health care is felt more
broadly than Americans might expect.[8]

THE COMMUNITY BENEFIT STANDARD:
A BRIEF LEGAL HISTORY

As noted above, nonprofit tax exemptions can be understood as a social contract
between the government and charitable organizations, but this contractual language implies more clarity of legal obligation than the community benefit standard has ever actually possessed. The standard's looseness reflects the time in
which it was written, following the creation of Medicare and Medicaid. As
responsibilities to care for elderly, poor, and disabled patients shifted from public hospitals and ad hoc charity care to a safety net of government-financed
programs, it seemed that the coverage gaps in US health care would close. As a

result, the IRS replaced its 1956 charity care standard for nonprofit hospitals with the 1969 community benefit standard.

The 1956 ruling stated that a nonprofit hospital must be "organized for educational, scientific or public charitable purposes," though "usually, the ground for exemption is that it is organized and operated for public charitable purposes." Teaching hospitals and research centers could qualify for a tax exemption on educational or scientific grounds, but the ruling's thrust was that a nonprofit hospital had to operate "to the extent of its financial ability" to serve patients "in need of hospital care who cannot pay for such services," either in part or in full.[9] Thus charity care was a de facto requirement of nonprofit hospitals' tax exemptions.

The IRS's 1969 ruling explicitly "modified [the earlier ruling] to remove therefrom the requirements relating to caring for patients without charge or at rates below cost." In place of the charity care mandate, nonprofit hospitals had to meet two tests. First, they must operate with a nonprofit structure, a community board, and an open medical staff. Second, they must promote health in the community. But note how community was defined: A hospital's charitable purpose, its "promotion of health," must be "beneficial to the community as a whole even though the class of beneficiaries eligible to receive a direct benefit from its activities *does not include all members of the community, such as indigent members of the community*, provided that the class [of beneficiaries] is not so small that its relief is not of benefit to the community." The clearest indicator of a broad-enough community benefit was "operating an emergency room open to all persons" even if the hospital admitted only paying patients to the main facility.[10]

This change in IRS rules can be read in two ways. The first reading accepts the language of the 1969 ruling as wiping away all traces of the earlier charity care standard. The 1969 ruling explicitly states that the "promotion of health" is a per se charitable purpose similar to "the relief of poverty and the advancement of education and religion," each of which is sufficient for tax-exempt status under US law. Nonprofit universities and religious congregations do not have to demonstrate that they relieve poverty to maintain their tax exemptions; the "charitable purposes" of advancing education and religion suffice. Likewise, a nonprofit hospital's promotion of health in a community could also suffice. Beyond operating an open emergency room, a hospital could fulfill this charitable purpose with health fairs, medical screenings, and wellness programs not specifically targeting poorer people. On this reading, the 1956 ruling that nonprofit hospitals relieve poverty by providing uncompensated care "to the extent of [a hospital's] financial ability" unfairly required them to serve dual charitable purposes.

The second way of reading the community benefit standard is that it was "begotten from motives of public policy," not precise legal categories. I borrow this pregnant phrase from the 1956 IRS ruling, which cited the US Supreme Court's holding in *Helvering v. Bliss* that the liberal tax exemptions that non-profit organizations received early in the twentieth century "were begotten from motives of public policy, and are not to be narrowly construed."[11] Courts have been similarly cautious in not construing the 1969 ruling too narrowly. In this case the changed policy landscape was the 1965 passage of Medicare and Medicaid. With hopes that patients' need for uncompensated care would decrease dramatically, the community benefit standard afforded nonprofit hospitals ample leeway to answer two questions: what constitutes "promotion of health" and what defines "community" in an era of public insurance. However, in light of numerous legal challenges and vocal public criticism over the decades, nonprofit hospitals' answers to these questions have not been well-received. Legal scholar John Colombo describes how first the IRS and then the courts abandoned the community benefit standard's "promotion of health" legal test. There is now a "promotion of health plus" standard, Colombo concludes, with the plus a tacit renewal of the old charity care mandate.[12]

Which reading of the community benefit standard is correct? The promotion of health test did not, in fact, establish a new legal definition of charitable purpose in health care. Instead, the 1969 standard should be viewed as a promissory note, written by the IRS and redeemable by nonprofit hospitals as they developed new forms of distinctive service. In this second and better reading, the community benefit standard was not a sea change in US law that released nonprofit providers from expectations of uncompensated care. It was a work in progress from the start, an experiment to define in practice what health care for the benefit of the community should look like after the implementation of Medicare and Medicaid.

Since that time, the community benefit standard has been transformed by an evolving policy landscape. Most importantly, the Emergency Medical Treatment and Active Labor Act of 1986 required all full-service hospitals to stabilize and treat any patient who presents at their emergency room regardless of ability to pay. Today all nonprofit and for-profit hospitals with emergency facilities must provide uncompensated care, so the difference made by a nonprofit hospital having an open emergency room has largely disappeared. Furthermore, because nonprofit and for-profit hospitals both use educational, wellness, and outreach

programs to drum up business, the other differences made by community benefits programs have lessened, too. Not surprisingly, for-profit hospitals started
asking whether nonprofits should retain their tax-exempt privileges if for-profit
hospitals match their required community activities. As this criticism grew and
as the number of uninsured and underinsured Americans continued to grow,
there was a way for nonprofits to make a clear difference—by providing higher
levels of charity care than for-profit hospitals. Thus recent state laws mandating
that nonprofit hospitals provide a "reasonable" or "minimum" amount of charity care—from 3 percent to 8 percent of annual revenues or operating costs—
aim to ensure that nonprofits distinguish themselves by offering measurably
higher rates of uncompensated care.[13]

The priority given to uncompensated care and Medicaid shortfalls on the
new Schedule H suggests an emerging consensus that nonprofit organizations,
and religious providers in particular, have a special public duty to fill the gaps
in the health care safety net by providing mandated levels of charity care.
Although there is agreement that nonprofits should provide distinctive benefits,
there is disagreement about what those benefits are and whether the distinction
should be qualitative or merely quantitative. We can tease out these differences
by listening to the moral conceptions of community benefits voiced by religious
providers and their critics.

COMMUNITY BENEFITS AS SOCIAL CONTRACT

The legal evolution of the community benefit standard signals considerable public distrust of nonprofit hospitals. Critics allege that these hospitals are not serving their mission and values and are hiding behind the vagueness of moral ideals.
As nonprofit hospitals have merged into large corporate health systems, there is
a growing sense that they have lost their way. A good example is the argument
made by Jack Hanson of the Service Employees International Union's (SEIU)
Hospital Accountability Project. Hanson affirms the "social contract" between
government and nonprofit health care organizations. The basis of this contract
is twofold. It started early in the twentieth century with the initiative of "private
charities and beneficent groups around the country . . . to establish community
hospitals to provide medical care to families unable to pay for doctor visits at
home." It culminated in the "recognition of [these hospitals'] charitable missions and of the important public benefits to be gained" as governments granted
them "special status as nonprofit organizations" with tax exemptions.[14]
Although not codified as law, this moral history, Hanson argues, makes public

expectations of uncompensated care a fixture of nonprofit hospitals' legal status and the financial benefits that flow from their tax exemptions.

Hanson posits a health care social contract based on implicit agreements that escape the letter of the law. These social agreements about the public value of charity care and the fairness of granting tax exemptions in return are congruent with the history of health care as a social good described in chapter 3. Hanson appeals to these underlying moral expectations throughout his argument. For example, he cites Stan Jenkins, a county Board of Review official who challenged the tax-exempt status of Provena Covenant Medical Center in Champaign-Urbana, Illinois.[15] For Jenkins, the tax exemptions enjoyed by nonprofits are "*a gift from public treasuries*," and the "term 'charitable purpose' as applied to a community hospital . . . connotes *an involved, proactive presence both in their communities in general and with respect to their patients in particular.*"[16]

This gift economy—gifts from the public treasury in exchange for gifts of community presence and service—induces specific obligations. As Hanson puts it, by granting a tax exemption to nonprofit hospitals, the "government is, in effect, contracting to purchase from the private sector goods and services that are supposed to address important community-identified needs." Two obligations follow. First, nonprofit hospitals' community benefits should "equal or exceed the value of [their] preferential tax treatment." Second, nonprofit hospitals must involve "community members in the community benefits planning process." Hanson concludes that currently "the public is not getting what it is paying for from nonprofit hospitals," and he singles out religious providers as particularly in breach of their social contract.[17]

I am keenly sympathetic to this democratic notion that the people granted tax exemptions and are due accountability in the use of foregone public funds. I welcome Hanson's brief moral history of the health care social contract that grounds his argument and recommendations. Other critics simply presuppose the existence of a quid pro quo agreement that nonprofit hospitals are to provide uncompensated care in exchange for tax exemptions. Such arguments enjoy bipartisan support as public officials at the federal and state levels have struggled to address the health care access and billing problems faced by many Americans.

Sen. Grassley, for example, has led the federal push. In 2007, he invoked a New Testament parable to spur nonprofit hospitals to publicize their uncompensated care policies. These "policies shouldn't be hidden under a bushel. They should be in the light for all to know and see."[18] In a draft proposal of remedies to the community benefit standard, his staff appealed to the virtue of stewardship to demand more charity care from nonprofit providers: "Congress should meet its responsibilities of being good stewards of the taxpayers' monies and ensure that in exchange for the billions of dollars given in tax breaks, nonprofit hospitals do in fact provide concrete benefits to the community, especially to the most vulnerable in our nation."[19] These moral appeals to shining charity care policies and congressional stewardship of tax revenues, however, substitute for legal citations of statutes and regulations. The lack of explicit legal authority is clear in Grassley's call to replace the 1969 community benefit standard.[20]

At the state level, Illinois attorney general Lisa Madigan (D) proposed the most stringent law in the country on the amount of charity care required of nonprofit hospitals. The Tax-Exempt Hospital Responsibility Act, which stalled out in committee, called for an 8 percent minimum of annual operating costs to be spent on charity care. In Illinois charity care is defined as excluding reimbursement shortfalls from *all* public programs. Unlike Schedule H's provisions, not even Medicaid shortfalls count. Hinting at gospel parables of abundant loaves, Madigan charges, "Hospitals that benefit from huge tax breaks have an obligation to give back to the community. Right now, hospitals that receive entire loaves of bread for free are handing out crumbs when it comes to providing health care to some of the most vulnerable Illinoisans."[21] The case for nonprofits' charity care responsibilities has a sounder legal footing in Illinois' 2003 Community Benefits Act and in Article IX, Section 6, of the Illinois Constitution, which states: "The General Assembly by law may exempt from taxation only . . . property used exclusively for agricultural and horticultural societies, and for school, religious, cemetery and charitable purposes."[22]

Even as an 8 percent charity care minimum is deemed fiscally impossible by all but the most dedicated safety-net hospitals, no public official in Illinois is proposing the 100 percent commitment that might be inferred from an "exclusive" use of nonprofit property for "charitable purposes." Here we return to the vagueness of charitable purpose at the center of the community benefits debate. In place of the legal vagueness that has characterized the community benefit standard, the social contract model inserts two principles: (1) uncompensated care is the essence of charitable purpose in health care, and (2) there should be rough parity between the dollar value of a nonprofit hospital's tax exemptions and the dollar value of its losses on the cost of uncompensated care. Advocates for the social contract model of community benefits fill in the interpretive gap separating the 1969 ruling from these principles through appeals to moral history, public virtue, and gospel parables. That nonprofit hospitals view these arguments as moral arm-twisting, not legal reasoning, is unsurprising.[23]

COMMON GOOD: TWO VERSIONS

In Catholic health care the moral basis of community benefits is common good, a concept that is notoriously difficult to define, especially in a pluralistic democracy. Furthermore, the common good is a multilayered concept so that priorities shift as the evaluative field expands or contracts organizationally, geographically, and socially. For example, the common good within an organization (fair pay and benefits for all workers) can conflict with the common good outside the organization (more charity care for poorer patients). I have heard this complaint voiced eloquently by union members in religious health care organizations.[24] They note the economic tradeoff between free and discounted services for the poor and higher wages and benefits for low-income hospital employees. For their part, service workers resent it when the common good is applied to external charity care but not to internal economic justice. In fact, both concerns are central to Catholic teaching about the common good.[25] Understanding how such tensions get resolved is the first step in assessing common good as a model of community benefits.

The common good has at least two components: the shared goals that people commit to with other people and the basic human needs that are met through networks of economic and social interdependence. Beyond these two components, Catholic health care leaders disagree about the exact location of the common good. Consider the contrast I heard drawn between a Jesuit and a Benedictine model of common good. A vice president for leadership development asked, "Does the community exist for the benefit of the individuals, or do the individuals exist for the benefit of the community?" A regional CEO developed this distinction in terms of the competing moral pulls of cooperation and sacrifice. In his words, "The Jesuits define common good as that we will band together our efforts so that individually each of us can do good. The Benedictine common good is that we will band together our efforts so that collectively as a group we can do good, meaning somebody might have to sacrifice. The Jesuit approach, and obviously this is a generality, . . . is no, no, no, we're not going to sacrifice. . . . The CEOs tend to define common good in Jesuit terms. Yes, we'll cooperate as long as we can do better." No doubt Catholic hospital executives who operate within conglomerate systems must decide when to sacrifice their hospital's priorities for the collective good and when to insist on mutual benefit. Despite the moral superiority accorded to the Benedictine common good here, the historical trajectory of Catholic social teaching has moved away from the idea that the collective good takes priority and that individuals must sacrifice on its behalf. Out of respect for the liberal commitments and institutions of modern democracies, the twentieth-century moral theologian Jacques Maritain relocated the common good from the binding ends that further the collective good to the enabling institutions that promote individual flourishing in common.[26]

This revised understanding was crystallized by the director of ethics at a Catholic system. In his words, the common good is an "infrastructure of well-being." In this model, community benefit serves as one of the ways to build the infrastructure of well-being in health care. The director of advocacy (from the chapter's epigraph) defined her organization's multifaceted "charitable purpose" as encompassing "healthy communities, community benefits, mission and ministry, and direct community investment." Here community benefits is considered one part of a strategy of promoting health throughout a community.

Parts of this strategy may take precedence at one time or another, and it is interesting to hear how some religious sisters with active leadership roles in Catholic health care describe the special significance of charity care, which they define more strictly than the IRS does. Invoking her organization's core value of justice, one nun affirmed the idea of a just minimum found in the social contract model of community benefits. In her words, "Giving what I am expected to [give] is justice. So I meet my tax exemption: That's justice, it's not charity. The next level is charity, and I think we've gotten back that understanding, that language . . . that over and above what is required, then that is the charity that we give." Another nun echoed this distinction between a contracted minimum and actual charity. Citing SEIU's scrutiny of community benefits practices as a help to her arguments, this mission leader pressed her colleagues to raise the bar. In her words, "Where the tire hits the road" in real community benefits is "in-kind donations and free services." For these sisters, meeting their obligation of community benefits requires more than providing uncompensated care up to the level of an organization's tax exemption. Community benefit extends the hospital's charitable work into building up an infrastructure of well-being out in the community.

Sister Carol Keehan, president of the Catholic Health Association, discussed this broader outreach in her testimony to the House Ways and Means Committee in 2005. Keehan recounted the work of Providence Health near the US Capitol. In addition to running a clinic in a local impoverished neighborhood, Providence Health funded a community center with a "nursery school, job and computer training programs, dance and karate classes." Clearly, the cost of the clinic fits the IRS definition of community benefits, but does the cost of the community center? In arguing that it should count, Keehan appealed to a fuller notion of common good as the proper basis and measure of community benefits. She claimed that we must "look beyond charity care" to "efficient" care delivery and "community-wide activity."[27]

Keehan raises three important questions related to turning the community benefit standard into an accounting standard of the financial losses that hospitals incur on uninsured and underinsured patients. First, are a hospital's financial losses on charity care an adequate measure of its social responsiveness to people's unmet needs? Second, does requiring hospitals to accept a minimum amount of annual financial loss on uncompensated care promote cost savings throughout the health care system? Third, how far does the safety-net provision of charity care in hospital emergency departments and clinics advance the goal of support- ing healthy communities? These objections introduce the shortcomings of a community benefit standard that takes charity care as the singular expression of charitable purpose. I address the three objections in order, beginning with the questionable equivalence between a hospital's financial losses and the health needs of the underserved.

COMMUNITY BENEFITS AS COMMON GOOD: BEYOND MANDATED LOSSES

A hospital's losses on uncompensated care are clearly related to its uncovered patients' health needs. But we have to distinguish between losses and needs in debating what should count as community benefits. The main questions in the public debate have been quantitative. For example, a common question is whether hospitals when calculating financial losses should count the costs or the charges of uncompensated care, knowing that uninsured patients are typically billed at full charges while insured patients tend to pay only costs. Schedule H uses costs. Another question is whether hospitals' community benefit losses should include bad debts—the bills that have been sent to patients who cannot or will not pay. Schedule H excludes bad debts. Finally, should legitimate losses include the shortfalls between a hospital's costs and the reimbursements it receives from Medicare, or should these losses be restricted to the shortfalls in Medicaid and other means-tested programs? Once again, Schedule H opts for the more restrictive definition but allows hospitals to estimate the community benefits portion, if any, of their Medicare losses and their bad debts.

On each of these questions, the IRS followed CHA's guidelines exactly.[28] Certainly, standardizing community benefits accounting and adopting stricter definitions will prompt nonprofit hospitals to distinguish their community benefits from their for-profit competitors. This goal is admirable, but the community benefit standard should not be reduced to a series of accounting questions meant to guarantee that nonprofits meet some contracted level of uncompensated care. The basic problem with the social contract approach to community benefits is that it makes financial losses *the* way to justify quantifiable tax breaks. Certainly, the numbers have to be watched to ensure that nonprofit hospitals provide community benefits commensurate with reduced public revenues. Yet a strict social contract model will intensify the disputes between nonprofit hospitals and their critics while limiting potential solutions to a zero-sum framework of economic and moral tradeoffs.

The economic tradeoffs arise in the context of today's competitive health care market in which 50 million Americans lacked insurance prior to the ACA. In this environment, every full-service hospital must attract high-paying patients to offset its legally required losses on uncompensated care in the emergency department. The more that community benefits are restricted to charity care, the more that nonprofit hospitals will have to pursue capital-intensive growth to attract patients with private insurance in order to maintain enough revenue flow. This economic tradeoff makes community benefits, when limited to charity care, a tool for filling gaps in an increasingly expensive system instead of a tool for investing resources in the kinds of efficient health care delivery and community health initiatives for poorer patients called for by Sister Keehan.

The moral tradeoff arises when the autonomy that religious nonprofits expect is reined in because they are judged to have fallen short of their tax-exempt obligations. The more that government officials demand greater sacrifices for the collective good, the more that religious providers will contest this meddling with their mission. Such skirmishes over who defines charitable purpose in health care will make for bruising legal battles without addressing Keehan's first proposal that community benefits include more than hospitals' losses. Simply put, if community benefit equals mandated losses, then the system will be too brittle to serve the basic needs and shared purposes at the heart of a common good conceived as an infrastructure of well-being.

COMMUNITY BENEFITS AS COMMON GOOD: COST-EFFICIENT INNOVATIVE CARE

Now consider Keehan's second community benefits proposal: pioneering cost-efficient protocols for delivering quality care to vulnerable populations. The perspective of a physician who became the chief executive officer of a medical group in a west coast Catholic system provides interesting insight partly because he equated business values with mission values so baldly. In his words, what distinguishes "our ministry, or our business," is our "market leverage" as the "big dominant system" in town. Owning several hospitals, a medical group, and a health plan, the organization can innovate on the community's behalf. As the medical group CEO put it, "There's a recognition that integrated systems of care have some value in today's market—that coordinating the care [through a hospital system, health plan, and medical group] is beneficial for each patient and, of course, more efficient as far as the cost of health care in today's society."

As an example, this executive focused on his medical group's diabetes registry of nine thousand patients and its proactive approach of calling patients in for frequent visits, monitoring their vital statistics, and doubling the number of patients meeting clinical outcomes for better health. This intensive outreach by social workers, pharmacists, nurses, and physicians raised the medical group's expenses. In addition, the parent organization invested heavily in information systems. Despite these added costs, however, the health plan's projected savings on catastrophic care was enough to fund a "small quality incentive or a bonus" for the medical group's doctors and staff to reward them for their increased work on preventive care.

The diabetes registry was not only a business success. In terms of mission, the initiative served the organization's goal of "ministering to the poor," who experience more complications with diabetes. In terms of values, the decision to invest in new information systems met the cost-saving imperative of the core value of "stewardship." The integrated business structure also "incentivizes," in the CEO's words, the core value of "compassion," while doing "justice" by compensating the staff. I find this seamless mixing of business language and mission language rather jarring, but also challenging to the assumption that mission is always at odds with margin. To put it bluntly, the money changers and the numbers crunchers are needed in the temple if the goal is beneficial and efficient ministry to poor and vulnerable patients.

This executive did not state which of the expenses of the diabetes registry should count as community benefits. Presumably the outreach to diabetics meets the "promotion of health" test, suggesting that a portion of the social workers' and pharmacists' pay should count as community benefits. What about the millions invested in information systems to facilitate the registry? Do they count as community health improvement services? Turning from costs to savings, should the physician and staff bonuses count as community benefits expenses? If the health plan passes some of its savings onto its enrollees, should this financial benefit be factored into the balance sheets of public gains paid for with lost tax revenues?

Behind all of these accounting questions, there lurks a more basic reason for skepticism. What if the diabetes registry and community outreach further strengthen this religious provider's market dominance, advancing its financial interests? Restricting the community benefit standard to a charity care mandate would make it much easier to draw bright lines around allowable community benefits, and such a sacrificial model fits the Benedictine conception of common good. The problem, however, is that it rewards financial losses without reducing social costs or improving health outcomes. By sapping hospital resources, it may even discourage more efficient delivery of health care that transforms the current system and meets the pressing needs of underserved patients in the community.

COMMUNITY BENEFITS AS COMMON GOOD: COMMUNITY ACTIVITIES

I turn, finally, to the community benefits resulting from community-wide activities. A Catholic system operating across the country has launched a network of community coalitions in the rural and urban locations its hospitals serve. The nun-turned-mission leader who presented this healthy communities initiative focused on spirituality, solidarity, and social justice, or what she called making "God's presence known."

The sister's description of spirituality emphasized the importance of building lasting and trusting relationships inside and outside her nonprofit organization. To cite Catholic ethicist David Hollenbach, the common good shows chiefly in the goods that are made possible only *within* relationships among people.[29] In this fashion the conversations about mission and values inside religious health care organizations can manifest the common good in action. The sister described facilitating executive-decision sessions by drawing participants into shared reflection on mission and values before tackling contentious tradeoffs. In her words, "I don't worry so much about the outcome, even if we make mistakes, and we will. It will survive—the 'common thing'—because of the integrity of the people and the good that comes."

This elusive "good that comes" has significance beyond senior executives debating big decisions. One of the most hopeful extensions of the good that comes out of dialogue among people working in solidarity was the effort to build coalitions of local leaders and citizens to advise hospitals about the health needs and health assets in a community. The process of building a coalition was long and costly. It began with local leaders but included a professional facilitator and funds for transportation, babysitting, and the other logistical expenses of citizen participants, all paid for by grants from the sponsoring health care organization. With the steering committee in place, the citizen participants met to set priorities, map assets, employ needs assessments, analyze strategies, and develop action plans to remove local access barriers or to target problems ranging from childhood obesity to gaps in dental care. Of course the good that comes out of these relationships depends on who shows up at coalition meetings. One coalition made keeping developers out of Amish property their first priority, to the dismay of the local hospital CEO. How is this "healthy community," he asked the mission leader nun, who reportedly replied, "Shut up, it will come later. . . . What's health? Housing's health. Safety's health. We've got to expand, and that takes patience."[30]

Asking local people about existing health care needs and enlisting them in putting unused assets to work in lowering access barriers reorients community benefits toward the values of solidarity and subsidiarity. First, solidarity expands as local people meet to identify health needs and assets in their communities. As the nun put it humorously, "We have to get away from this maternal image that we can do it. But we can facilitate a heck of a lot." The more that hospitals facilitate the proactive definition of community benefits by local people, the less that community benefits will be dictated by hospitals' financial losses. Second, subsidiarity deepens as community members take action, partnering with the hospital and local government to mobilize resources and concern. This devolution of authority to the lowest possible social level was symbolized for the nun by the discovery in one locality of different dialectics of Spanish spoken by various immigrant groups and the need for "coalition[s] within a coalition" to give all people voice and "develop leaders."

Which parts of this initiative should count as community benefits? Only the organization's grants to launch the coalitions and fund their health programs? Does the goal of preserving Amish property count? If a local church uses its van to transport patients during the week, can a hospital count the funds given to the religious organization for gas? Instead of starting with technical questions like these, policymakers should first ask two broader ones. What, in addition to financial losses on uncompensated care, should count as community benefits? How much money, time, energy, risk, and reputation can nonprofit organizations afford to expend in the absence of credit and support from a better-targeted community benefits policy?

The examples discussed above suggest answers to these questions. Community benefits policy should advance two priorities: (1) pioneering cost-effective treatment protocols for chronic disease management among vulnerable populations and (2) engaging stakeholders in defining local community health needs and cooperating to deliver health care more equitably and accessibly. Both initiatives require significant financial, strategic, and motivational investments. Here the internal and the external dimensions of the common good interact positively. Serving the external common good through innovative treatment protocols and through community identification of needs is helped along by the internal common good, the "common thing," the "good that comes" out of commitments to examine and debate shared mission and values. Here religious providers have something distinctive to offer: deep experience with internal deliberation about mission and values that generates financial, strategic, and motivational investments in improving access, lowering costs, and extending quality care to vulnerable populations in order to meet neglected needs. Let me be clear. I am not suggesting that only religious providers engage in mission dialogues. Nor am I proposing that their mission budgets count as community benefits expenses.[31] Rather I highlight the dynamic of *mission in motion*, which presses beyond the task of meeting the quid pro quo of a social contract to the goal of building up the infrastructure of well-being integral to a common good.

COMMUNITY BENEFITS AS COVENANT: JEWISH COMMITMENTS AND CAVEATS

Jewish interviewees in my study also expressed their dissatisfaction with the numbers game of community benefits. As observed by a Jewish professor of public health who oversaw community benefits at a Catholic system, "Where the whole community benefits field has gone astray in a regulatory sense is that it's mainly an accounting definition." Jewish interviewees and hospitals brought other commitments to the discussion, too. Notably, they raised caveats about the CHA approach to community benefits, which has become the regulatory standard of the land. These caveats begin with Jewish skepticism about the universalism and spirituality presupposed by a Catholic conception of community benefits as common good.

By universalism I mean two things. First, Catholic health care organizations celebrate service to the whole community. Historically, Catholic hospitals were founded to serve Catholic immigrants and any Catholics who felt excluded from or proselytized to by Protestant charitable institutions. Today these organizations dedicate their service to all constituencies.[32] Second, the broad applicability of CHA's community benefits guidelines is an instance of the universalism in

Catholic social teaching. The vision of a public square where citizens can debate common values is central to the natural law traditions of papal encyclicals and bishops' letters. These documents are directed not only to Catholics but to the whole society. Catholic universalism is expressed both in the goal of serving everyone equally and in the belief in common moral values.

By spirituality I mean something more elusive. This spirituality is clearest in Catholic providers' identification of their history, culture, and service as a ministry infused by Jesus Christ's healing spirit. As observed by a self-described "little-B baptist" legal affairs director who worked for a Protestant health care system before joining a Catholic one, Catholic health care is distinguished by its sacramentality. "Through ritual, through structure," he noted, mission takes on a life in his organization in a "more visible, more present" way. One example of the mission made tangible is a commissioning ritual at a West Coast system where new lay executives are anointed with oil and charged with carrying on the founding nuns' gifts of service, their charisms. Another manifestation of this Catholic form of spirituality is the Church's language of healing body, mind, *and* spirit. Even the ongoing dialogical reflection on mission and values within these organizations is seen as an expression of spirituality in Catholic health care.

Jewish interviewees shared both humorous observations and serious reservations about the professed universalism and spirituality of Catholic health care. The ubiquity of prayers at the start of meetings in Catholic organizations was frequently noted. "It makes Jewish people very nervous when you start praying," commented a Jewish communications official, "because they're afraid that when you get to the end you're going to go 'in Jesus's name, amen.'" This Jewish executive and a nun also shared a fascinating exchange over the term spirit as they discussed the challenges of merging their Jewish and Catholic health systems. Their disagreement—really a misunderstanding on the nun's part—turned on whether the history and identity of Jewish hospitals express Judaism as a religion or Judaism as an ethnicity. As discussed in chapter 2, the Talmudic injunction to heal even on the Sabbath elevates the duty of lifesaving care to the highest priority of health care justice. In addition, Talmudic scholars stipulated that Jewish communities must support a physician and a surgeon. In the nun's mind, these covenantal commitments to provide excellent care to patients and research and training facilities for Jewish physicians and nurses stemmed from ethnic rather than religious motivations. For her the religious quality of a health care organization inheres in the "spirit" in which it offers care, while the communications official emphasized that, for Jews, "spirit" connotes praying together in church, at the bedside, or in organizational meetings. Jewish commitments to justice in delivering excellent medicine encompass compassion for patients, too. For the nun, however, more is required—both a spirit of self-sacrifice and a communion of spirits—to fulfill religious mission in health care. This exchange underscores the difficulty of aligning such Christian categories as spirit, mission, ministry, and charity with the historical motivations and contemporary commitments of Jewish hospitals.

Admittedly, these two sets of religious motivations and models of healing differ subtly. But Protestant ethicist William F. May has taught us to attend closely to the images that people use to characterize their moral responsibilities. Images, in his words, "provide a comprehensive ordering of life—an interpretation of role, metaphysical setting, and institutional context—that makes moral behavior seem more like a rite repeated than a puzzle solved."[33] The image of the common good as an infrastructure of well-being makes the institutions and roles in which people participate deeply formative of their capacities and virtues. It also entails wide-ranging responsibilities for other people's needs and flourishing. The spirituality and universalism of a Catholic common good are once again clear. The result is a model of community benefits that can seem practically unlimited in its reach and demands.

A Jewish covenantal model of community benefits is more delimited in several respects. First, in a covenantal model, duties of justice, not aspirations to charity, are primary. Second, a covenantal model is fully consonant with the idea of concentric circles of moral responsibility, with special duties to some groups of people giving way to a general expectation to care for the broader community. Finally, the sharing of duties among different institutions, each with its own covenanted obligations and sphere of expertise, further narrows, for example, the scope of a hospital's responsibilities for medical care when compared to the government's responsibility for the health care safety net. This emphasis on putting duty first, and specifying the duties that different professionals and institutions have, makes a covenantal model of health care more delimited than a common good model, especially one characterized by universality of obligation and spirituality in intent.

The historical tendency of Jewish hospitals toward excellence in teaching and research and their founding goals of serving Jewish immigrants and providing medical training and hospital privileges to Jewish physicians and nurses reflect these twin covenantal themes of duties of expert health care and special obligations to particular constituencies.[34] A covenantal model of community benefits also gives reasons to object to a charity care mandate and the IRS's adoption of CHA's reporting guidelines.

The director of government relations at a Jewish hospital system with an 80 percent Medicaid and self-pay patient population, for example, objected to the intense focus on community benefits by public officials. She agreed that every hospital "should open [its] doors, everyone should be providing uncompensated care" at the level her hospital does. Yet, in her words, charity care is such "a nineteenth-century concept." Providing free or discounted care to people through emergency departments is "very inefficient, and it's a very bad way of distributing resources." She called the charity care legislation at the state and federal levels a "red herring." Certainly, she said, "we would feel better if everybody kicked in [an equivalent share of uncompensated care], but it's not an answer to the problem of the uninsured. . . . The answer to the uninsured is to insure people," with the government meeting its covenanted duty of guaranteeing universal coverage.

A second policy objection is that the moral calculus behind the CHA guidelines may do unintended harm to those hospitals currently providing some of the highest levels of charity care: urban safety-net hospitals.[35] The decisions to calculate charity care as costs rather than charges and to exclude bad debts from community benefits data are reasonable at first blush. Hospital charges are always negotiated down by private insurers and public programs, so counting the charges for uncompensated care is excessive. However, hospitals calculate the cost basis of their care using an array of expenses, including depreciation on their facilities. The older facilities of many safety-net hospitals lower their cost basis, making their losses on uncompensated care relatively small compared to the losses claimed by hospitals with newer facilities. It makes no sense to minimize the contributions of cash-strapped safety-net hospitals when calculating community benefits.

The exclusion of bad debt from community benefits has an equally good justification. Some patients fail to pay for their care, and these uncollected bills get counted as bad debts, one of the costs of doing business that every nonprofit and for-profit hospital faces. CHA's decision to distinguish nonprofit care by excluding bad debts from charity care has to be understood, however, in light of Medicare regulations and Christian theology. Medicare rules require hospitals to establish every patient's eligibility for uncompensated care prior to billing. If this eligibility cannot be established, then the unpaid costs of care must be listed as bad debts. This position is echoed by Christian theology in which charity depends on the giver's intent, not just the recipient's need. Theologically, bad debt is not charity care because, when the care was given, there was no explicit charitable intent of not expecting payment. Uncompensated care cannot therefore be made charitable after the fact, after one realizes the patient's inability to pay, because the spirit of giving was absent at the start. Financially, however, what distinguishes the act of giving care to someone who does not pay due to indigence or to shirking? The care is uncompensated in either case.

Making matters more difficult, safety-net hospitals face significant challenges in meeting these Medicare (and CHA) charity care guidelines. When a young gunshot victim is patched up at an emergency department only to discharge himself soon afterward, the chances of obtaining the financial information to qualify him for charity care are slim. Likewise, immigrant patients and transient populations served by urban safety-net hospitals may be unwilling or unable to document their finances, hindering hospitals from qualifying them for charity care. So starts the process of sending a bill to an invalid address, beginning the slide toward bad debt and removing the cost of this care from the new Schedule H. Once again, safety-net hospitals, which provide disproportionately higher levels of uncompensated care, are likely to have their community benefits under-counted compared to hospitals with a stable patient base.

These objections notwithstanding, the CHA guidelines do help standardize the reporting of community benefits data by different hospitals. Counting costs, not charges, deflates the exaggerated figures claimed by some providers. Separating out bad debts requires hospitals to try harder to qualify self-pay patients for free or discounted care before they are billed full charges. Excluding Medicare reimbursement shortfalls, but not Medicaid, rightly reflects the payment imbalance built into public programs to "care" for the elderly but to "aid" the poor, the disabled, and those elderly who require nursing home care. As the IRS compiles standardized data on which nonprofits have the highest rates of uncompensated care and Medicaid shortfalls, the widely disproportionate shares assumed by nonprofit hospitals will further reveal the inequities in US health care.

Yet the data will not capture the stories on the ground, a frustration of interviewees who argued that social justice considerations in building a fairer health care system take precedence over the sideline issue of how exactly to count community benefits. Social justice is contextually sensitive as a social contract is not. A social contract model of community benefits is a zero-sum numbers game: Do the losses on uncompensated care equal the value of a hospital's tax exemption, or do they measure up to its charity care mandate? Social justice presses beyond the numbers to investigate where individual patients live and how they access services. A key question of social justice is, how does a patient's social location help or hinder access to quality care?

The chief financial officer of a Jewish system noted that, in choosing to remain at its inner-city facility instead of moving to the suburbs, his system traded in its covenant with the Jewish immigrants who built the neighborhood for a covenant with the African Americans and Latino immigrants living there now. Although the founding community left, the founding purpose of serving a marginalized community persists. This covenantal obligation is increasingly stretched, he reported, by the large number of suburban poor who also seek care at this hospital instead of at the hospitals in their suburban neighborhoods. This situation speaks to the "common bads" in US health care. The flipside of an infrastructure of well-being, common bads result from an infrastructure of inequality wherein some people's privileges for excellent care are purchased, in part, by commanding so many resources that little is left for others.[36] When the suburban poor feel alienated by the upscale facilities near their homes, cultural divisions are added to the geographic and economic distances in US health care. It is easy to understand why, and morally justifiable that, this CFO envisions a time when his hospital may have to turn away self-pay suburban patients to serve the local patients more immediate to its current covenant with the poor.

THE FUTURE OF COMMUNITY BENEFITS: THE BETWEEN AND THE CONNECT

As implementation of the Affordable Care Act proceeds, what relevance does the decades-old community benefits debate still have? Is the United States entering a new era in which the old rules no longer apply? In the wake of the implementation of Medicare and Medicaid, the IRS foresaw a sharp decline in the need for uncompensated care and therefore released nonprofit hospitals from their charity care obligations. The 1969 "promotion of health" test did not, however, establish a new definition of charitable purpose in nonprofit health care. This chapter has reviewed the three competing models that shaped the contours of community benefits as the legal standard evolved in response to shifting public policies and to the practices of religious providers, led by the Catholic Health Association.

These models are not abstract ideals. They have taken concrete form in public policies governing community benefits and in the delivery structures built by nonprofit providers. This moral history sustains social norms of service, inclusion, and shared responsibility. Political philosopher Michael Walzer, from whom I borrowed my three principles of distributive justice in part 1, offers another observation about social goods that applies here. Part of what makes such goods as health and health care "social" is that they assume recognizable moral structures and shared meanings in particular societies. In Walzer's words, "goods with their meanings—because of their meanings—are the crucial medium of social relations; they come into people's minds before they come into their hands."[37] It is difficult to wrap our minds, let alone our hands, around social goods as complex as health and health care. If we take them piecemeal, however, and consider, for example, the community benefits that nonprofit health care providers are both legally required and socially expected to provide, then these implicit moral structures and shared meanings come clearly into view.

Each of the community benefit models presupposes its own distinct moral structure, helping to explain the fervor of the public debate. With these moral structures now before us, several promising conclusions emerge. First, there is broad bipartisan and interfaith agreement that nonprofit hospitals have public responsibilities, especially to poor and vulnerable people. This social norm challenges reform agendas that cast individual Americans back on their own health care resources. Second, religious appeals to common good and covenant are not restricted to denominational statements that rarely see the light of day (see chapter 2). Instead, religious nonprofits have made these moral ideals concrete by debating their practical significance and by building delivery structures in their image. Finally, the practical expression of these religious norms adds to the public understandings of health care that Americans share. They are part of the diverse ethical inheritance of people living in the United States. Secular worries about the self-enclosed morality of religious groups do not apply here. Instead, public discussion is enriched when people identify and claim the full range of moral traditions in the nation's ethical inheritance and hold one another accountable for making one's public arguments, along with the underlying secular and religious reasons, as transparent as possible.[38] As Americans debate health care reform, it is vital that they take stock of the shared values invested in the social good of US health care not only through public policy and government funding, but also through the philanthropic initiatives of mission-driven nonprofit organizations.

If we take seriously religious nonprofits' commitments to covenant and common good, then a social contract model of community benefit is inadequate by itself. Instead, in charting the future of community benefits, social responsiveness should take priority over social responsibility. Comprehensive in scope and basic in obligation, social responsibility is the purview of government. Local in scope and contingent in obligation, social responsiveness is the charge of nonprofit providers. Jewish covenantalism reinforces this division of duties. The collection of taxes from citizens and businesses commits government to the social responsibility of ensuring a fair and effective health care system and safety net. The ACA reduces but does not eliminate the need for uncompensated care. Americans whose individual mandate is waived for financial hardship and immigrants who cannot participate in Medicaid or the state insurance exchanges will still seek uncompensated care. In addition, in states that refused to expand Medicaid in 2014, millions more low-income Americans will remain dependent on uncompensated care. In other words, the "nineteenth-century concept" of charity care will remain with us, even as the ACA should reduce unmet need and uncovered expense. It is worth emphasizing that these gains result from more than increased public spending. The ACA facilitates a broader sharing of social responsibility in health care financing through its individual mandate, its employer mandate on firms with over fifty full-time workers, and its insurance regulations on community rating, coverage denials, payment caps, and medical loss ratios. Thus individuals and businesses, not simply the government, are called to meet their covenantal obligations for a more socially responsible health care system.

The projected decrease in uncompensated care in the wake of full implementation of the ACA may obviate the push for charity care mandates, but there is a more compelling reason to reject them. Requiring nonprofit hospitals to lose a fixed percentage on charity care will escalate the competitive race after paying patients. Overall health care costs will rise as providers double down on high-technology, procedure-driven care delivered in facilities with all of the amenities. To return to the chapter's epigraph, community benefits "has to be put in a different kind of lane," particularly for religious providers. That does not mean excusing nonprofit providers from the public accountability of the social contract model. Nonprofit hospitals should be able to quantify annual community benefits at the level of their tax exemptions. The challenge is matching the accountability measures to the goals of a wiser community benefits policy. Of the three moral models, I believe the common good is the best way to retool the policy mechanics of community benefits.

Social responsiveness requires building an infrastructure of well-being in the areas served by a nonprofit provider. It means connecting to communities through needs assessment and collaborating with organizational partners to respond to local problems and local opportunities through mission-driven linkages and innovations. In this way social responsiveness is more dynamic and transforming than social responsibility.

Although she did not use the term social responsiveness, the nun who described the healthy communities coalitions gave a clear portrait of its purpose. She related a typical story: "You bring a kid into our emergency room with pneumonia. Not a problem. We can have that kid back on her feet, all fixed up, and she goes back to an apartment with no heat. Are we health care providers?

No. I mean who's responsible?" Summing up the challenge in a pithy epigram, she continued, "That's the between and the connect." Where nonprofit providers can make the biggest difference is recognizing the spaces in "between" existing health care services and then helping "connect" patients to community services and relationships that sustain better health. Conceived as "the between and the connect," community benefits should not be reduced to the social responsibility of guaranteeing care to uninsured patients. Otherwise the distinguishing trait of the more innovative nonprofits, their social responsiveness, will be discouraged.

Using Schedule H as a roadmap, we can project the likely detours and plot a route for the future of community benefits.[39] The ACA may or may not decrease the top category of financial assistance for uncompensated care and Medicaid under-reimbursements. The expected decline in uncompensated care may be offset by a growth in Medicaid enrollees. If, however, financial losses in these two areas decline, there will be a strong tendency to shift this portion of hospitals' tax exemptions to such community health-improvement services as health fairs, medical screenings, and education programs. Too often these familiar initiatives focus more on marketing hospital services than connecting people to disease-management programs in community health centers, backed by the supportive presence of parish nurses and the trusting relationships among neighbors that encourage healthier habits and reduce return visits to the hospital. Another detour would be if nonprofit hospitals simply increased cash and in-kind donations. Annual community benefits reports once included laundry lists of all the employee hours volunteered and other nice but random acts of assorted people working for a large organization. Pressuring providers to simply do more quantifiable community benefits will not yield the integrated strategies for improving the infrastructure of well-being in US health care.

This chapter outlined two priorities that should govern community benefits policy in the coming decades: (1) enlisting community stakeholders to partner on behalf of more equitable uses of local health care assets and (2) pioneering cost-saving protocols for delivering quality care that improves the health of poorer populations. Currently nonprofit hospitals cannot claim the costs incurred or the savings produced through these activities as community benefits proper.

To its credit, Schedule H signals the importance of the first priority. Part 2 of the form requests data on nonprofit hospitals' community-building activities in housing, economic development, coalition building, leadership development for community members, and many other areas. In the words of the mission-leader nun, "What's health? Housing's health." Hospitals can "facilitate a heck of a lot" by building healthy community coalitions. Encouraging hospitals to work beyond the walls of their facilities is not enough by itself. For example, they should not receive credit for investing in just any housing initiative, only those that address an identified community-health deficit. Protecting Amish housing from developers would not qualify as a matter of course, but it might if the disruption of Amish communities exacerbated mental illness in a demonstrable way. Admittedly, translating this deficit principle into a workable policy framework will be difficult. The first step is conducting health needs assessments that clearly profile the patient populations in a nonprofit hospital's service area. That involves scouring the terrain for underserved groups, meeting with community representatives, and identifying the community assets that foster health and the persistent barriers that inhibit health. Annual community benefits reports should spotlight not only the successful mobilization of community assets and hospital resources, but also the remaining health challenges that exceed the hospital's capacity. Here the social responsiveness of nonprofit providers operates within the broader social responsibility of governments.

A more daunting accounting challenge is calculating the dividends returned by innovative treatment protocols that reduce costs and improve outcomes for people with chronic diseases and other health concerns that disproportionately affect vulnerable populations.[40] Schedule H offers no help here, though help might come through the accountable-care structures encouraged by the ACA. Although the ACA restricts accountable care organizations (ACO) to Medicare, the idea is translatable. In the ACO structure, groups of physicians collaborate with hospitals and other providers to manage care with earlier interventions, greater continuity, and better integration. Any savings on the reduction of expensive procedures, hospital readmissions, and catastrophic care are shared between the payer and the ACO. Nonprofit hospitals could take their ACO savings and weight them in terms of their percentage of Medicaid and uninsured patients. This figure would approximate the cost savings achieved through better treatment protocols for poor and vulnerable patients, a figure that could be added to Schedule H as direct community benefits.

Turning these proposals into enforceable policy is a task for others. Still we can identify the principle, the means, and the goal of a better community benefits policy. The principle of social responsiveness justifies two new categories of community benefits: the cost of community coalitions and community-building activities that address demonstrable health deficits, and the expense of innovative treatment protocols that pay back in lower-cost care that also improves the health outcomes of vulnerable populations. Together these strategies can enhance the means of an infrastructure of well-being that promotes the goal of healthy communities across the United States.

A wise community benefits policy puts social responsiveness before social responsibility. In both the covenant and the common good models, governments collect taxes from citizens and businesses, and government is therefore charged with social responsibility. By contrast, when governments forgive the taxes of nonprofit providers, they recognize that these organizations have unique capacities for social responsiveness, but that does not make them into an arm of government. Dividing the labor in this way does not excuse nonprofit providers from their obligations of uncompensated care. Rather it expands their community benefits options toward a more socially responsive transformation of US health care.

NOTES

1. Salamon, *Partners in Public Service*, 33–52.

2. Schlesinger and Gray, "Nonprofit Organizations and Health Care," 378, 379, 385.

3. Some critics argue that nonprofit hospitals should provide community benefits above their tax exemptions to match the profits, taxes, and community benefit services at for-profit competitors. See, for example, Nicholson et al., "Measuring Community Benefits."

4. Dubler, "Introduction," 9. For comparison, see McCormick, "The Catholic Hospital," 651. McCormick opposes the shift from the physician-patient focus of bioethics to the public morality of health care ethics.

5. The IRS released a discussion draft of Schedule H in June 2007: www.irs.gov/pub/irs-tege/form990scheduleh.pdf. For the final draft, see www.irs.gov/pub/irs-tege/f990rschh.pdf.

6. Internal Revenue Service, *IRS Exempt Organizations Hospital Compliance Project*, 84.

7. Principe et al., "The Impact of the Individual Mandate," 231.

8. American Hospital Association, "Fast Facts on US Hospitals: 2010," www.aha.org/research/rc/stat-studies/fast-facts.shtml (accessed Sept. 27, 2012).

9. Internal Revenue Service, "Revenue Ruling 56–185."

10. Internal Revenue Service, "Revenue Ruling 69–545," my italics.

11. Internal Revenue Service, "Revenue Ruling 56–185."

12. Colombo, "The Failure of Community Benefit," 32–37.

13. For an overview of state laws and initiatives in Texas, Rhode Island, Pennsylvania, and Illinois, see US Senate Committee on Finance—Minority Staff, "Tax-Exempt Hospitals," 9–10.

14. Hanson, "Are We Getting Our Money's Worth?" 396.

15. Japsen, "Provena Files Appeal over Tax."

16. Hanson, "Are We Getting Our Money's Worth?" 401; Hanson's italics.

17. Ibid., 398–99, 404.

18. Grassley, "IRS Report Shows Non-Profit Hospitals Often Provide Little Charity Care."

19. US Senate Committee on Finance—Minority Staff, "Tax-Exempt Hospitals," 4.

20. Ibid., 3.

21. Madigan, "Madigan Proposes Two Bills."

22. Constitution of the State of Illinois, article IX; cited in the proposed "Tax-Exempt Hospital Responsibility Act," HB5000, Section 5(b)2.

23. Becker, "Charity with an Arm Twist."

24. Catholic theologian Charles Curran criticizes many Catholic hospitals' resistance to unions. In his words, "It is a grave understatement to say that Catholic hospitals have not supported and encouraged unions" ("The Catholic Identity of Catholic Institutions," 95).

25. The US Catholic Bishops' *Economic Justice for All* names the priority of basic services for the poor and the necessity of fair wages and benefits for workers as integral parts of the common good: 20, 24 (§86 and 103).

26. Maritain, *The Person and the Common Good*, 52–55, 63–65.

27. Keehan, "The Tax-Exempt Sector."

28. Catholic Health Association, *A Guide for Planning and Reporting Community Benefit*, 31–33.

29. Hollenbach, *The Common Good and Christian Ethics*, 8–9, 41–42.

30. Regarding the social determinants of health, Daniels et al. write, "Health is produced not just by having access to medical prevention and treatment, but, to a measurably greater extent, by the cumulative experience of social conditions across the life course" ("Justice, Health and Health Policy," 38).

31. I disagree with DeBoer that the "religious purpose" of serving mission and values by religious hospitals qualifies them for tax-exempt status ("Religious Hospitals," 1558–59).

32. Dolan, "Social Catholicism,"196–97.

33. May, *The Physician's Covenant*, 20.

34. Katz, "Paging Dr. Shylock!"

35. Unlike urban safety-net hospitals, rural critical-access hospitals are typically excluded from legislative charity-care mandates. See Illinois's proposed "Tax-Exempt Hospital Responsibility Act," § 35; and US Senate Committee on Finance—Minority Staff, "Tax-Exempt Hospitals," 7.

36. Hollenbach, *Common Good and Christian Ethics*, 189.

37. Walzer, *Spheres of Justice*, 7.

38. I take the notion of a diverse ethical inheritance and the norm of democratic accountability for religious and secular reasoning from Stout, *Democracy and Tradition*, 5–6, 10.

39. For a discussion of my recommended changes to Schedule H, see Craig, "Religious Health Care as Community Benefit," 324–25.

40. Chronic disease prevention "aimed at improving nutrition, physical activity, tobacco use, and related lifestyle behaviors are likely to have the greatest effect on slowing the annual increase in health care costs" (Shortell, "Bending the Cost Curve," 1223).

Chapter 5

Assessing Market-Driven Reforms
ECONOMY WITHOUT SOLIDARITY

> I spent the first twenty-five years of my career working on the idea that health
> care should be competitive. It will respond to market forces if we just figure
> out how to tweak the circumstances. Just set up some market forces. . . . Now
> I start with the idea that health care is a public good and a scarce commodity.
> So as a result, we have a social responsibility to try to deploy it in a way that
> reaches as many people as possible.
>
> Regional chief executive officer, West Coast Catholic health system

R ELIGIOUS HEALTH CARE PROVIDERS have to compete in the health care marketplace while serving their mission and values. Sometimes religious values can help sell a provider to patients, and marketing departments happily promote the sense of trustworthiness and compassion that many Americans associate with religious commitments. At other times mission-driven services pull resources away from investing in the latest technologies and newest facilities that attract privately insured patients to profitable service lines. In the parlance of religious providers and their critics, mission can enhance margin, but mission can hurt margin, too. Over the past several decades, many religious providers have merged in order to compete with other health care conglomerates and to earn large enough margins to cover the cost of their mission-driven care. A few statistics from Catholic health care providers illustrate the trend. In 2010, there were 630 Catholic hospitals in the United States concentrated into only 56 Catholic health care organizations.[1] Over half of those hospitals were owned by the eight largest Catholic systems, of which the three biggest ranked third, fifth, and eighth among US hospital systems by total revenue.[2]

Describing the competitive pressures to invest and grow, a mission leader from one of the big three Catholic systems raised the mission-versus-margin question. Mixing metaphors of a protective cloth and a competive sport, he asked, "To what extent can we stretch this Catholic fabric to fit the new world of economics? The dollars you need to do a certain ministry is a whole different ballgame of dollars that weren't needed in the past." There is also the challenge of maintaining a broad enough base of insured patients to cover the losses on uncompensated care. "We've had this problem with some of our major hospitals," he admitted. "If you are suddenly the dumping ground—the 'charity hospital'—what happens to your competition, your access to capital, and your future? It is quite possible that fidelity to Catholic social teaching in our economic environment could put you out of business." These stark words came from a priest who lived and breathed his organization's mission.

The business challenge for religious health care administrators is how to navigate the market pressure of needing to "get big" in order to survive while remaining faithful to mission. Policymakers ask a different question: Why has this consolidation not yielded the typical savings of increased scale? The regional chief executive officer quoted in the chapter's epigraph voiced one possible answer: We need to "set up some market forces." Increased scale cannot lower costs by itself. Other competitive pressures must also be brought to bear—on consumers to shop around for better price and higher quality and on providers to innovate new ways of delivering excellent care at a lower cost.

The first attempt to inject market forces into US health care led to the era of "managed competition." Under President Bill Clinton's proposed 1993 Health Security Act, large regional and corporate alliances of insurers would act as consumers, using their market power to pressure provider organizations to reduce costs and raise quality. Provider organizations would respond by paying their physicians to steer patient care away from expensive tests, procedures, and specialist visits and toward wellness, prevention, and chronic disease management. The resulting cost savings, supplemented by new sources of funding, were to have provided coverage for all Americans.

In the Clinton plan the new market forces would have operated at the macro level as large insurance alliances and provider organizations competed in a regulated marketplace designed to take advantage of their size. Conservative opponents argued that this managed structure of health care competition would cause a bureaucratic nightmare of rationed services, waiting lists, and red tape. Although conservatives offered alternative proposals, including some of the building-block reforms of the Affordable Care Act,[3] they mostly dragged their feet in favor of the status quo.

The conservative opponents of the Health Security Act are today's market reformers, and now they have no interest in the status quo. Not only do they decry the absence of market forces in US health care, but they also see managed competition as a half measure that would have increased the power of big insurers and big providers at the expense of consumers and physicians. Market reformers seek direct health care markets, where individual consumers can demand value and efficiency and where individual physicians are rewarded for delivering better care for the money. Market reform has to be assessed as a positive reform agenda. Americans should welcome the goal of a more responsive and rational delivery system, and putting health care decisions more in the hands of purchasing consumers and enterprising physicians might help contain costs and improve quality.

These values of economy and care are both essential to health care reform. Examining the market reforms already at work in US health care, however, we find that they have not served another equally important value—solidarity. This missing value of solidarity explains why the regional CEO, the one-time believer in market forces, changed his mind. Through dialogue sessions about mission and values inside his organization, he came to see that US health care is never simply a "scarce commodity"; it is simultaneously a "public good." Understanding this tension is critical in assessing whether market reforms can make US health care more efficient, competitive, transparent, and responsive—the market values championed by its proponents.

THE WHEELS COME OFF THE
HUB-AND-SPOKE SYSTEM

It is important to distinguish market reform from trends in the health care industry. With or without market reform, US health care is shifting away from the hub-and-spoke model of twentieth-century American medicine. Chapter 3 described how the federal government concentrated its construction, research, and training funds on teaching hospitals and community hospitals, making them the hubs of an increasingly specialized delivery system. Acute care and medical technology were located at the hospital hubs. Specialists radiated out the spokes to the primary care physicians lining the rim. This hub-and-spoke image suggests wheels of health care spinning merrily all across the United States. In fact, the picture was never that pretty, and in recent decades, the wheels have really started to come off.

Observing US health care from the outside, what strikes the eye is the proliferation of facilities, including new hospitals and outpatient services. It takes a journey inside a major health care organization to grasp the more fundamental shift afoot. The change is not only toward more variety of services in more places but also away from the centralizing role of the community hospital in coordinating care. These centrifugal forces include the following: (1) the expense of operating a full-service hospital, (2) the consolidation of the health care industry, (3) the diffusion of technology out of community hospitals, and (4) the competition from physician-owned specialty hospitals and outpatient facilities.

The chief organizational development officer at a midwestern Catholic system described the systemic challenge created by the legacy of "primary care, secondary specialists, [and] tertiary facilities." Pointing at his system's flagship general hospital, bristling with acute care towers, he joked, "We've got this big tertiary care piece over there that needs to be fed. You've got to organize to feed the beast." General hospitals are expensive because of all of the staff, infrastructure, and technology required to provide comprehensive acute care. Medicare's initial cost-plus payment system was a boon in meeting the fixed costs of running general hospitals. Cost pressures began in the 1980s when Medicare implemented its diagnosis-related group (DRG) payment system. In assigning a fixed fee for thousands of diagnoses, Medicare gave hospitals new incentives to limit patient stays. As a result, occupancy rates in hospital beds declined.[4] Then as new health care options began springing up across suburban America, community hospitals faced intense competition for the surgical procedures, diagnostic imaging, and other technology-intensive services that were their bread and butter. The development officer summed up the challenge succinctly: "A lot of the delivery system depends on volume, and the kind of volume [in community hospitals] is getting to be people who are self-pay and Medicaid over commercial pay."[5] In this economic environment, "People have to be sick for the system to be well. So what's wrong with this picture?"

The expense of running general hospitals in an era of declining payments and growing competition has led to the second trend of nonprofit hospitals consolidating into health care conglomerates. The mergers can run horizontally in combining multiple hospitals, or they can run vertically in employing physician practices, partnering with physician-owned facilities, and even offering health insurance plans. By spreading the expense of acute care hospitals across multiple locations and by diversifying into different service lines, most hospitals in the United States have remained afloat, and new ones continue to be built. Ironically, as hospital organizations invest in physician practices and outpatient facilities, even more of their traditional business migrates out the door.

These system-level changes have altered the internal workings of religious providers, too. For example, the pressure to consolidate has weakened one of the cornerstones of Catholic social teaching—the principle of subsidiarity. Subsidiarity encourages decision making at the level of the smallest social unit capable of exercising effective authority. A nun who directs mission at another midwestern Catholic system commented, "I've always embraced the teaching that says push decisions down to the lowest possible level," adding wryly, "except maybe in my own family." By devolving power to the local level, more people have opportunities to develop leadership skills and virtues, and decisions are more likely to be responsive to community needs. The principle of subsidiarity requires building the local common good first in order to serve the common good overall.

A retired chief executive officer of a Pacific Northwest Catholic hospital bemoaned the loss of subsidiarity in his former organization. As a non-Catholic chief executive, he appreciated how his organization's layered authority gave him the latitude to decide which services met the community's needs and whether patients could receive emergency procedures at odds with Catholic teaching. He noted regretfully, "Today in our system it's just the opposite. Authority is being sucked upward. Purchasing, medical records, admitting, billing, collections, and accounting" are all performed at the state level. While conservatives decry the centralization of power in government bureaucracies, it is important to recognize the growing power of corporate bureaucracies in US health care. Consolidation and centralization can cut operational expenses, potentially freeing up funds for patient care if the savings are not absorbed by administrative salaries. But saving money at the corporate level does not serve community responsiveness if centralization prevents people lower down in the bureaucracy from developing the right skills, authority, and feel for the communities where they deliver health care.

Market reformers are also critical of the consolidation of the health care industry. They want to replace "big box" hospitals with smaller, focused, physician-owned clinics and hospitals. As a result, they are much more supportive of two other trends: the diffusion of technology out of community hospitals and new competition from physician providers.

Forty years ago community hospitals housed nearly all of the advanced technology in US health care. In 1973, the federal government mandated states to develop certificate of need (CON) laws. These laws created an oversight process of first establishing that a community already had new health care needs before authorizing the "certificate of need" required for hospital construction and purchases of advanced technology. The aim was to curb health care inflation by avoiding redundant facilities and equipment and their duplicate capital and staffing costs. The federal mandate for CON laws ended in 1987, and fourteen states have repealed their laws, while others have scaled theirs back.

The retreat of CON laws is a major factor behind the diffusion of technology. Magnetic resonance imaging, computed tomography, da Vinci surgical robots, and other expensive devices have spread out across the suburbs into new community hospitals and the diagnostic imaging centers and hospital competitors owned by physicians. Even the chief operating officer of a Catholic hospital system was happy to see the county CON boards eliminated in his midwestern state. At the county level, he argued, party politics can determine who wins and loses in the new-construction and technology race. In his words, "County borders are party political boundaries. They are not the way that most people think about receiving and delivering their health care services." With one of his system's hospitals located two miles from a county line, he criticized the county board's stringent test of community need as harmful to the hospital's employees and local economy. "People would drive two miles to the McDonald's in [the next] county to have a hamburger. Surely they would make that drive for their health care. So strict county limits put a burden on [our hospital] which had already made an investment in the community and wants to make an additional investment now."

According to this interviewee, CON laws fit the hub-and-spoke model of the community hospital as medieval fiefdom, but not the wild west of market competition. "Absent putting walls around the county with appropriate guard stations and a moat," he said, "you couldn't keep the patients in and couldn't keep the competitors from putting their forces at the border's edge." When I asked if CON laws could be adapted to the more fluid terrain of today's health care marketplace, this executive allowed that community needs could be determined by boards of health professionals at the state or national level. "Now if we could save tens or hundreds of millions of dollars on health care resources, I would be comfortable with that approach." But he added that competition from new providers can lower prices, too, potentially more than offsetting the short-run expense of duplicate capital investment in new construction and technology if inefficient providers are driven out of business in the long run.

One major source of new competition has been the shifting relationship between hospitals and physicians. In the hub-and-spoke model, physicians are the entry point into the community hospitals where they have admitting privileges. With clusters of high-tech services increasingly located outside the central hub, physicians have more referral options, while hospitals remain beholden to their admitting physicians. One of the lightbulb moments in my study came during an interview at the same Catholic system run by the free-marketeer

COO. The director of human resources described the careful path she has to tread with the very physicians who are building, or threatening to build, their own imaging centers and specialty hospitals: "What's so screwy in the health care system is that we depend on the physicians to admit their patients here. So how abrasive can you be with the very people who are sending patients to your door? The hospital walks a tightrope because physicians are our biggest customer. Without them we don't have a patient. Patients cannot admit themselves to a hospital." Anyone who has been a patient in a hospital will likely find this statement jarring and yet also confirming. We think that hospitals are organized for patient care, so the patient is the customer. But hospitals live or die based on their "biggest customer," their admitting physicians. Keeping doctors happy frequently demands aggressive investment in the technologies and facilities with which to ply their trade.

Two crucial points follow from recognizing the changing relationship between hospitals and physicians. First, under the hub-and-spoke system, the lone community hospital functioned something like a community oversight board in performing two functions—determining which investments were most needed and redirecting resources from profit centers like cardiology and surgery to money losers like mental health services and chemical-dependency treatment. Today, the community hospital has lost considerable oversight authority. Its role is more that of a supplicant, having to entice physician referrals and sometimes partner with physician-owned competitors to avoid bleeding away all of the lost revenue required to "feed the beast."

Second, although the opponents of market reform dislike calling patients "consumers," the term has transformative potential. It is especially important to recognize that in today's US health care, physicians too are consumers. The physician orders tests, prescribes medicine, schedules procedures, refers to specialists, and so on. There is no health care consumption without a physician order, and in a fee-for-service payment system, physicians have incentives to consume more services. In this reality, insisting as market reformers do that patients should have the consumer's usual powers of pricing out and selecting their services might push US health care to become more patient-centered and more cost-effective.

In fact, the decline of the community hospital may be just what the doctor ordered. Many observers of US health care argue that the infrastructure for delivering care must shift away from acute care toward wellness, prevention, and chronic disease management. This claim highlights another structural problem in the hub-and-spoke model. The spokes connect only in the hub. In other words, specialists practice their discrete areas of medicine with little to no coordination across the spokes. In theory, the community hospital once served as a place for integrating care, though when administrators redistributed resources from high-profit specialties to money losers, physicians' turf battles could be so intense that they inhibited cooperation.

Market reformers argue that physician-owned facilities are the future of integrative care. As health economist Regina Herzlinger puts it, "The need for some form of integration arises because the health care system is organized around the providers of care and not around the needs of users of care." Addressing the most common, debilitating, and expensive health problems facing Americans—diabetes, heart disease, hypertension, asthma, and mood disorders—involves physicians spread out all around the hub-and-spoke wheel. Market reformers advocate "focused factories" that cluster teams of diverse specialists in providing holistic care for one complex condition.[6] These focused factories promise to lower average costs by scaling up one set of services instead of offering the community hospital smorgasbord. Providers that achieve the best health outcomes for the money would attract more patients whose consumer-directed health plans require them to pay more of their bills. As successful providers gain market share, competitors would try to improve on their innovation. Thus market efficiency would seem to lead to higher-quality care for the sickest patients at a lower cost to the overall system.

Assessing market reform as a positive agenda for reorganizing US health care, its most significant potential contributions include (1) the replacement of employer-sponsored group health insurance with consumer-directed health plans and (2) the decline of community hospitals in favor of physician-owned specialty hospitals and outpatient services. Next I examine the prospects for consumer-directed health care and physician entrepreneurship, comparing the economic values championed by market reformers with the fuller visions of good health care found in the missions and core values of religious health care nonprofits.

RELIGIOUS VALUES IN
A CHANGING MARKETPLACE

The shifts toward consumer-directed care and physician entrepreneurship are both well under way. On the insurance side, premiums for family coverage nearly doubled (97 percent) from 2002 to 2012.[7] In response the percentage of covered workers choosing the lower average premiums of consumer-directed health plans has jumped from 4 percent in 2006 to 19 percent in 2012.[8] On the provider side, there has been an explosion of hospital-physician competition as can be seen in the growth of physician-owned specialty hospitals from 127 in 2006 to 265 in 2010.[9] This hospital-physician competition has helped fuel a capital investment boom in new construction and technology.[10]

As religious providers respond to market trends, they have to balance economy with care and solidarity. All three values map onto the mission and value statements of religious providers. Economy, or the quest for better value for the money, appears in the appeals to stewardship, creativity, and innovation that frequent these organizations' lists of core values. Care, or the devotion to healing patients as whole persons, shows in the importance of compassion, respect, and quality. Solidarity, or the readiness to share in other people's risks and costs, is seen in the commitments to common good, covenant, and justice and in missions of caring for the poor and the vulnerable.

As argued in chapter 4, the values of religious providers matter to the extent that they are "articulated" in an organization's operations and delivery structures. Using this standard of judgment, we can assess market reforms by comparing the delivery and financing structures generated by market incentives with those of religious nonprofits, which ostensibly serve a wider range of values than efficiency, responsiveness, competitiveness, and transparency. One virtue of this structural approach is that it moves beyond moral arguments from on high, in which abstract principles and values dictate ideal delivery systems. Descending into the complexities of the health care marketplace demonstrates that the value of economy is essential to any sustainable reform. Cost control must be part of whatever reform path Americans choose to take. Equally important, the silent partner to economy, the value of solidarity, must become clearer in the public's understanding of how US health care works and fails today.

Focusing on economy and solidarity, I argue two claims. First, to date, consumer-directed health plans and physician entrepreneurship have eroded the structures of solidarity that have operated implicitly in US health care. Second, contrary to the aim of market reform, the value of economy is frustrated by this erosion. Comparing market reforms to the structures of religious health care organizations challenges the efficiency and responsiveness of consumer-directed care and the competitiveness and transparency of physician entrepreneurship. Religious health care organizations have been reticent to draw these contrasts themselves, but bringing their articulated values to the health care reform debate can help Americans judge which organizational structures and policy reforms are likeliest to deliver quality care efficiently and fairly.

CONSUMER-DIRECTED HEALTH
CARE: HOW EFFICIENT?

Consumer-directed health care aims to give consumers more control over their health care dollars. Since 1997, US law has allowed high-deductible health plans (HDHP) to be paired with a tax-deductible savings account.[11] The deductible exposes consumers to the first several thousand dollars (or more) of their annual health care costs. The tax deductions and lower premiums aim to soften the blow. Although covered Americans may be wary of assuming this level of financial responsibility, HDHPs build on a central tenet of economic theory: consumer sovereignty. Simply put, individual consumers know their preferences and resources and are therefore best positioned to make two tradeoffs. In the context of their overall budgets, consumers can decide how much of their annual income to spend on the financial security of health insurance compared with other non–health-related goods. In addition, consumers will be wiser judges of how to allocate their spending on health services, wellness activities, and the other components of good health if they purchase most of their health care directly.

Consumer-directed care is meant to serve the value of economy in two ways. On the one hand, consumer choice can make US health care more cost-efficient. The more that consumers are exposed to their health expenditures, the thinking goes, the more incentives they will have to shift their priorities toward wellness and prevention and to shop for better prices on medical treatment. In this way consumer-directed care can tap into the calculating and negotiating power of consumer choice.

On the other hand, consumer choice can make US health care more responsive to individuals' judgments of value. Market reformers see these judgments as currently frustrated by third-party decision makers in three ways.[12] Employer-directed health insurance forces consumers to "choose" unnecessarily comprehensive policies. Big-box hospitals charge excessive prices to cover their massive overhead while collecting billions in public subsidies. Government price controls drive physicians away from poor areas, leaving expensive emergency care the only option. At issue here is not simply the high cost of third-party decisions. These decisions frequently protect the status quo, inhibiting innovative insurance plans and health care services better suited to individual consumers' preferences.

With the promise of consumer-directed care before us, it's useful to take up the two sides of market efficiency in turn. I start with the goal of cost savings (getting the money to go farther) before shifting to the goal of improved quality (getting better value, too).

Understanding how consumer-directed care might help with cost control returns me to the category question in the chapter's epigraph. Is US health care a scarce commodity or a public good? The director of ethics and mission at a large Catholic health care system wrestled with this question. On one hand, he began, health care is a "basic good like education and fire protection." It is basic to human flourishing because the good of health allows people to participate in family, work, leisure, and so forth. In a country with a vast health care infra-structure amply supported by public funds, it is deeply objectionable to exclude people from these basic services. On the other hand, he added, health care is also a commodity because "you have the right to shop around and buy the best product for you." In every health care system resources are limited. In the United States, people gain access to health care partly on the basis of their ability to pay. The abundance of some health care services over others is often the result of their profitability, too.

Then the conversation turned to uninsured patients whom the mission and ethics director called "bad consumer[s]." He continued, "They're accessing a commodity that is higher priced [in emergency departments], and how do we manage that uninsured person with this consumer-driven health care? How do we educate them to make better choices? That's playing the hidden game. If we say, well, we're not going to play that game, then we miss the opportunity to address the issue of the uninsured in a different way." This ambivalent embrace of commodity language jars with Catholic social teaching since Pope John XXIII that medical care is a human right.[13] It also softens the hard reality of seeking primary care in emergency departments. At the same time, the description of health care as both a basic public good and a scarce market commodity reflects the current organization of health care in the United States. The claim that health care is basic to many other goods and the fact that public funding covers half of US health care costs have been established in previous chapters. The commodity features of US health care show in the way that delivery priorities are set within the limits of scarcity operating in any health care system.[14]

Limits on health care resources—the number of caregivers, the amount of flu vaccine, the availability of diagnostic technology—are inevitable. Other nations manage this scarcity through public mechanisms of governance. For example, Canadian legislators set global budgets and then a health care bureaucracy of government agencies, oversight boards, and provider organizations prioritize the most cost-effective means to promote good health outcomes and quality of life. In the United States, by contrast, providers start with their own budgets and set their investment and delivery priorities with an eye to growing their annual revenues. Consumers have "the right to shop around and buy the best product," which gives providers economic incentives not to stretch their piece of the global budget as far as possible, but rather to grow annual revenues by investing in the most profitable service lines and attracting the better-paying patients. As a result, service profitability and market share are the key external drivers of US health care. It is little surprise, then, that health care inflation outpaces the rest of the economy as market pressures all run in the upward direction of expanding profitable services and enticing privately insured patients with costly amenities.

To their credit, market reformers view this organizational structure as lopsided. Market pressures cannot only run upward. They must also run downward by providing consumers incentives to reward quality care delivered at a good price. According to market reformers, this structural problem has its origin in the hybrid nature of US health care. Health care cannot be part public good and part market community; it must be all market commodity. With government paying half of the bills in US health care, the push for market efficiency should begin with public insurance programs, they argue. For example, in my home state the Healthy Indiana Plan is a HDHP for low-income enrollees that combines required monthly individual contributions with public subsidies to fund health savings accounts.[15] Rep. Paul Ryan's (R-WI) Medicare reform proposals go farther in redirecting public funding entirely toward premium support for private insurance.

What should we make of these proposals to bring consumer-directed health care into public insurance programs? Market reformers insist that they are not turning their backs on patients who are insured by Medicare and Medicaid. They argue quite rightly that treating US health care as a basic public good without acknowledging that it is also a scarce commodity, which must somehow be limited through priority-setting, will make the goal of universal access too expensive to attain. Furthermore, they predict, if health care is treated as a market commodity with a transparent price tag, then innovative providers will seek the potentially large profits to be earned through holistic chronic disease management to the benefit of poor and elderly Americans and at lower overall cost to taxpayers.

These promises of greater economy in US health care are very attractive, but there is a fatal flaw to the market-driven approach. A single-minded pursuit of economy at the expense of solidarity will fail to deliver the savings promised by market reformers, a problem that can be illustrated with examples of consumer-directed care cutting across class lines.

There was disagreement in a Jewish hospital system about the practicality of offering consumer-directed health plans to Medicaid patients. On one side, the CEO of a network of affiliated clinics supported health care vouchers for Medicaid patients to fund a health savings account. Rewards would include the power as paying customers to choose their own doctors. In addition, people who used their funds judiciously could bank their annual savings for future health care or possibly use them for other expenses. On the other side, the hospital's chief financial officer noted the difficulties of "penalizing" the Medicaid consumer and many Medicare consumers. If patients cannot afford a high deductible on their health care services, dunning late payments would do little to change their behavior. Health savings accounts funded by public money might help alleviate this problem, he acknowledged, but they would be difficult to arrange for those consumers who operate outside the banking economy. Most importantly, if health care is simply a commodity alongside all of the other commodities tugging at a poor person's limited resources, we arrive back at distorted economic incentives. Instead of the current incentive of seeking primary care at a hospital emergency department, the new incentive would be to postpone routine and preventive care (the better to use voucher money in other ways).[16] But the fact is that health care is a basic good in human life; it cannot be ignored forever. When a lack of regular care leads to poor enough health outcomes, people will eventually seek care. The longer they wait, the more expensive the care will be. Admittedly, care could be refused to patients who cannot afford the market price, but almost certainly the American public will still be paying the bills for emergency and critical care when they come due at the hospital—in this case because of a "rational" consumer preference for short-term savings.

Consider now patients with chronic conditions. The regional CEO quoted in the epigraph cites two effects of a move toward HDHPs with health savings accounts. First, the distance between the "haves" and the "have-nots" will grow. As the young and healthy opt for less comprehensive coverage and bank part of their annual deductibles, they will build "a war chest of money" for themselves. By contrast, patients with chronic conditions will "blow out their deductible every year" while facing higher premiums due to the adverse risk selection of being grouped with relatively sicker and older people. Any cost savings achieved by the young and healthy in foregoing or bargaining down the costs of their discretionary care will redound to them, but not to others. As a result, the economy promised by consumer-directed health plans weakens the solidarity built into large risk pools that combine the healthy with the unhealthy. The second effect is that the predicted cost savings of consumer-directed care will be less than advertised. The CEO notes that patients with chronic conditions will be "unresponsive" to a high deductible given their continuing needs for care. Because the largest portions of US health care spending cover the elderly and the chronically ill, the overall cost savings from consumer-directed care will be fairly small. In sum, not only will a lack of solidarity reduce the projected gains of greater economy, but people with the gravest health needs will likely see the costs of their care rise.

Consider, finally, patients with the time and resources to shop for discretionary care. A hospital foundation leader predicts that "we're going to a consumer-driven market where quality indicators and cost indicators are going to be readily available, and it makes everybody sit up and do better." One prerequisite for such an outcome is widespread dissemination of price lists and quality ratings. As a human resource director notes, however, "our finance people . . . couldn't give me a pricing list, so how is Joe Schmoe going to be able to figure that out?"[17] Transparent price and quality data are sorely needed in US health care. Driving this information out into the open would be an achievement, and angry consumers having to pay thousands of dollars or more in annual health expenditures might get the job done. There are so many providers, however, that data collection is a difficult task for all but the largest insurance companies. Moroever, the limited pricing data they provide lists prices in such wide ranges (e.g., one company might list the cost of one service as $500 to $700, and another company might list the cost of the same service as $450 to $800) as to be meaningless. Moreover, the consumer feedback that is currently collected applies only to superficial elements of provider quality, such as the demeanor of caregivers and the appearance of facilities. Accurate price lists and meaningful health outcomes will prove elusive so long as insurers and providers offer only estimated charges and superficial quality ratings aimed at growing their market share.

Given the cost-insensitive nature of health care for the poor, the chronically ill, and the elderly, it is a mistake to project the benefits of consumer-directed health plans on the basis of people who are well positioned by decent health, health coverage, and savings to learn prudence in their discretionary health care decisions. Many Americans may fit this category for much of their lives, but when a commodity is also a basic good and is amply funded by the public, there will be spillover costs whenever care is delayed or risk pools shrink. The Catholic concept of a "social mortgage" on private property applies here.[18] The relatively high insurance premiums paid by the young and healthy, the larger share of health care costs borne by big firms, the cost shifting of providers' losses on the uninsured and underinsured to private insurance payments,[19] and the redirection of community hospital revenues from profit centers like cardiac care to money losers like psychiatric care are all examples of the structures of solidarity that have operated implicitly in US health care. These structures have effectively "taxed" the benefits enjoyed by the most powerful consumers and successful physicians to make the basic good of health care more widely available.

These mechanisms for sharing in other people's health risks and health care costs impose what we might call a solidarity surcharge on the insurance premiums and medical bills that covered Americans pay. Market reformers are right that transparent pricing is needed to help everyone control costs. Transparency should also include informing consumers of their solidarity surcharges. Imagine a hospital bill that broke out the expenses for physician care and other services rendered. A final item would estimate the portion of the total bill that covers the cost of care for uninsured and underinsured patients. Insurers could do the same with their premiums. Such transparency might inspire ire or empathy, but at least Americans would understand how much they already share in one another's health risks and health care costs. One likely result of consumer-directed health care is that it will reward low-price providers who get ahead by discounting the hidden structures of solidarity from their bills because they do not provide care to uninsured or underinsured patients. Their personal gain will leave the social costs of unmet needs to more responsible competitors. Needless to say, this kind of market efficiency is not real efficiency. Instead I would encourage religious providers to put their moral authority to work in publicizing true pricing data, including a "solidarity surcharge," to teach Americans how much we already share in one another's health care.

CONSUMER-DIRECTED CARE: HOW RESPONSIVE?

Other scholars have noted that consumer-directed health plans disadvantage uninsured and chronically ill patients, so society's cost savings would be less than advertised in the event of wide adoption of this reform agenda.[20] My interviews add another reason to question consumer-directed care. In addition to cost efficiency, the proponents of consumer-directed care anticipate greater responsiveness from health care providers as consumers demand quality care that fits their judgments of economic value. Here the concepts of economic tradeoffs and consumer preferences are key. Once consumers confront the cost of their health care, they will face two new tradeoffs. First, there are the tradeoffs among different types of health care spending—for example, the different prices of preventive, chronic, and acute care. Second, there are the tradeoffs between health care and the other goods that consumers might prefer to purchase, whether other health-related goods like fitness and nutritious food or other competing necessities like housing and transportation. Market reformers predict that when faced with these tradeoffs consumers will prioritize healthy choices, wellness activities, and preventive medicine in their quest for better health for their money. Yet comparing market-driven delivery structures with the structures of religious health care organizations challenges this assumption.

To illustrate the deeper, unrecognized problem with consumer-directed care, we have to compare the narrow set of economic values championed by market reformers with the range of values professed by religious providers. The Catholic mission and ethics director introduced above offered an analogy that highlights the ambiguity between the term quality in the medical sense of good patient outcomes and quality in the economic sense of a desired product at an attractive price. He predicts that "consumers will look at quality like they do the airlines. They expect you to get them from point A to point B safely. United and Southwest do that. . . . What the consumer is looking for is the value. I'm flying Southwest. I don't need dinner, I just need peanuts. So I don't need what the hospital is trying to offer me [with its values]. I want value for my money, and are you giving it to me?" This analogy raises the question of how to balance the second part of efficiency—better value for the money—with the other values enshrined in religious providers' mission statements.

The time and resources that some religious health care organizations devote to mission and values seem like an inefficient diversion if patients prefer safe, effective treatment delivered as inexpensively as possible. This single-minded goal is attractive on one level. My interviews taught me, however, the importance of having different groups within an organization—financial managers, mission leaders, doctors, nurses, and service workers—represent competing values at the table. At least in organizations where debate and dissent are built into the structure, mission-driven dialogue increases the prospects that new delivery structures will be guided by more than financial viability and medical expertise.[21] Indeed, quality health care in the organizations I surveyed are often driven by shared mission rather than market share.

Consider the business strategy of a psychiatric hospital in a merged Jewish-Catholic system. As one of the few psychiatric hospitals to keep its doors open in recent decades, the organization survived by creating new programs for unmet needs, signing service contracts with the state, and generally "evolving to survive," in the words of its business director. Such flexibility and responsiveness are deemed inherent strengths of a market system, but the hospital's new business plan was not market driven. This religious provider decided to place psychiatrists in their primary care facilities to identify mental health problems earlier and to prioritize community-treatment options. This strategy has two disadvantages as a business strategy. It decreases average reimbursement per patient, and it steers patients away from the physicians with admitting privileges at the hospital. In the business director's words, "While we're staying busy, one of [our] focuses is how do you keep people out of a psychiatric hospital. In our advocacy role, what we're doing is working to advocate for more community-based services." He contrasted this approach with for-profit hospitals "doing assessments at mental health centers [and] doctors' offices and carting kids right into the psych hospital."

In this state's funding structure, hospital stays paid by Medicaid are reimbursed at higher rates than for any other payer. The economic incentive, therefore, is to treat patients in the hospital. Clearly this business plan would be untenable if the religious provider did not own community treatment centers, too, the result of a calculated growth strategy. Even factoring in the incentive of building patient numbers at the new centers and establishing relationships with potential users of the hospital's services, this early intervention approach is unjustifiable solely in terms of market payoff.[22] This raises a question: Are the goals of prevention and wellness, which serve both individuals and the community, likelier to be advanced by competition for market share or by commitment to mission?

The simple answer is the business director's answer: "The right thing to do is to help people stay out of the hospital." Implicit in his response are appeals to the values that have been taken up into the organization's business strategies. The implicitness is significant. Values do not stand out here as distant aspirational ends or mere public relations fodder. Instead they are built into the new delivery structures as a result of internal discussions of organizational priorities as they intersect with the needs of individuals and other resources in the community. This organization's core value of respect for human dignity puts a premium on promoting every patient's wellness and independence where possible. The core value of common good led the hospital to mix its resources with state and philanthropic funds to launch the community treatment initiative. By restructuring its care network and collaborating with community partners, the hospital launched the early-intervention initiative as a mission-driven, not a market-driven, effort to provide higher-quality treatment at a lower cost.

If this initiative had depended on the market incentives of consumer demand or provider profit, it would not have seen the light of day, a fact that exposes a defect in the supposed responsiveness of consumer-directed care: Giving providers economic incentives to respond to patients' judgments of value may not lead to good health care. Asking mental health patients to demand, in timely fashion, wellness and prevention services presumes a diagnostic acuity about one's situation and a discerning inventory of gaps in treatment options that are simply implausible. It is hard to imagine patients with almost any serious condition who could demand services not yet in existence. Without a push from the consumer side, however, what will steer market-driven providers away from remunerative, if less effective, treatments? As reported by the business director, for-profit providers in his state were still adding beds in their psychiatric hospitals rather than building community treatment centers. This economically rational but socially irrational decision will likely prompt future cuts to Medicaid mental health reimbursements.

The blunt instrument of government price controls is one of the chief complaints made by market reformers about the current health care system. Organizing health care as a public good, they charge, inhibits the responsiveness of market-driven innovation. As we have seen, however, responsiveness did not flow from market innovation in the case of the psychiatric hospital; it resulted from the coordinated action of a mission-driven nonprofit serving a range of values. Both the individual needs and the community assets had to be brought to light by a more penetrating vision than the market preferences of consumers and the market opportunities of providers.

At their best, dialogues among stakeholders representing the different values in a religious provider's mission can serve as a promising source for sustaining and rebuilding structures of solidarity in the face of shifting health care markets. The challenge for religious providers is to remain distinctive in the face of immediate market pressures. Offering care with a compassionate touch is insufficient. Drawing on ethical conceptions of common good means looking beyond the payoffs of acute care and the security of proven cash flows in order to partner, not simply compete, with local organizations bound implicitly in community care.

PHYSICIAN ENTREPRENEURSHIP:
HOW COMPETITIVE?

The other side of consumer-directed health care is physician entrepreneurship. In the proliferation of services out of community hospitals into specialty hospitals, imaging centers, and outpatient facilities owned partly or wholly by physicians, we see dramatic changes in health care delivery. I focus on physician-owned specialty hospitals (POSH) in examining how competitive and transparent physician entrepreneurship is likely to be. Although one never hears the acronym (a rare exception in the acronym-packed jargon of health care), most physician-owned specialty hospitals are POSH in their amenities and bottom-lines.

Debates about POSHs have been so heated that even the definition is contested. Fending off my questions about hospitals in his system, a government-relations director, who criticized the creeping individualism in health care, denied having any specialty hospitals in his Catholic system. For him "a specialty hospital is a clinical inpatient service that doesn't have an emergency room."[23] This definition fits ambulatory surgery centers but not the new heart hospitals, which typically have emergency rooms. What links all of these new facilities is their delivery of one set of specialized services. As noted above, Herzlinger praises these "focused factories" for their technical proficiency and economic efficiency.[24] Facilities dedicated to one type of care, say, for heart surgeries, can be used to perform more procedures by a team of highly skilled specialists who are motivated by financial investment and personal pride in the hospital.[25] How, one may wonder, could this efficiency and quality not translate into better care for the community through market competition?

Like the criticism of consumer-directed care, critics have focused on a more obvious objection to POSHs that masks an issue with deeper structural implications. The familiar criticism is that specialty hospitals engage in unfair competition. While supporters praise specialty hospitals for their market segmentation by type of procedure, critics allege market segmentation by type of patient. Because physicians choose either to admit patients to their own specialty hospital or to the community hospital where they have privileges, there are charges of cherry-picking patients with the best insurance, the most profitable diagnoses, and the least acute conditions.[26] Two features of US health policy justify these worries. Medicare's DRG payment structure sets fixed fees per diagnosis, so profits are made on patients with less severe conditions and no chronic complications. Patients requiring longer stays or intensive care lose money for hospitals. Those losses are compounded by the federal requirement of emergency treatment. Ambulatory surgery centers without emergency access have no legal requirement to treat uninsured patients, who are more likely to present with acute or chronic conditions.

Concerns about the unfair competitive advantages of POSHs led Congress to halt Medicare payments to those built between 2004 and 2006. In October 2007, the Centers for Medicare and Medicaid Services revised its DRG rates by adding a "severity" modification to reward hospitals that treat more acute and chronic patients. While this change reorients physician owners' incentives toward treating sicker patients at their own hospitals, it does nothing to prod specialty hospitals without emergency rooms to accept the uninsured.

The specialty hospital phenomenon raises two different questions, dependent on the questioner's degree of belief in the market as an instrument of reform. The true believer asks, If incentives to treat the healthy and the wealthy are the product of government policies, then why not remove any policy that interferes with market competition? The Medicare DRG structure and the EMTALA access law both frustrate a free market. Providers cannot name their prices or require payment for all services rendered. Yet eliminating the cost savings of DRGs and the safety net of emergency care would be intolerable as things stand today. We would lose the economy generated through DRG constraints and the minimal solidarity implicit in mandated access to emergency departments. Again, values must be built into structures, in this case the structures of federal policy. These implicit values illustrate why arguments for a pure market in health care are ideological. Health care markets will always be shadowed by policy structures, and a pure health care market would have too many gaps to sustain public support.

The more serious question is this: If policy adjustments can stop unfair competition, then does the prospect of increased quality, efficiency, and transparency in the patient care provided by specialty hospitals make them a straightforward gain for community care? Most supporters of POSHs make this argument: Fair market competition between specialty hospitals and community hospitals will improve quality, efficiency, and transparency.

Consider the experience of a midwestern Catholic system that partners with a physician-owned heart hospital. Having an emergency room and having adopted its parent system's charity care policy, this hospital has seen its percentage of uncompensated care rise from 3 percent to 9 percent of revenues. The physician owners already treated more of the acute cases at their own facility than at the system's nearby tertiary hospital, so the DRG severity revisions only helped this specialty hospital's finances. The doctors also rotate through the rural hospitals in the parent organization's statewide system, extending care outside the urban area served by the flagship community hospital. Using protocols developed for the new specialty hospital, the main hospital achieved the same improved patient outcomes as the cardiac center. Both hospitals reduced the number of expensive surgical interventions, arguably due to earlier intervention and preventive care.

This rosy portrait of one POSH suggests that market incentives can drive better care all by themselves.[27] This example must be considered, however, in light of the larger trends in health care markets, and specialty hospitals have several marks against them. One is the tendency to locate POSHs in middle- or high-income neighborhoods. Consider my city of Indianapolis, where every new specialty facility is located in the suburbs. In addition, POSHs focus on such remunerative areas as cardiac and orthopedic care, once major revenue streams for community hospitals. As capital flows to suburban facilities, more inner-city and rural patients may be left out of their high-quality care, while the community hospitals serving those patients struggle to "backfill" their revenue streams.

It makes a great difference that my sample heart hospital is part of a large system. Its charity care policy is the system's policy, its service to rural communities goes through the system's critical access hospitals, and its improved protocols benefit the system's flagship hospital. Take these internal organizational structures of solidarity out of the story, and the pursuit of better patient care at specialty hospitals is no longer as clear a benefit to community care. More importantly, the strengths ascribed to specialty hospitals by their defenders—their independence from big-box hospitals and their direct responsiveness to consumers—are complicated in this case by the structured cooperation between the specialty hospital and the community hospital. It is difficult to base policy on one example, but this one cautions against allowing entirely freestanding specialty hospitals and supports requiring every specialty hospital, even those that lack an emergency room, to provide uncompensated care.

The legislators who wrote the Affordable Care Act took a more aggressive step toward limiting the potentially unfair competitive advantages of POSHs. Section 6001 of the ACA denies Medicare reimbursement to any new or expanded POSH to which physician owners refer their own patients. Effectively, existing POSHs will not be allowed to expand, and no new POSH will be built given the dependence of all hospitals on Medicare payments.[28]

PHYSICIAN ENTREPRENEURSHIP:
HOW TRANSPARENT?

The public debate over POSHs has focused on charges that physician owners refer profitable patients to their own facilities. Once again, a deeper issue has gone unnoticed. In addition to the revenue streams new hospitals extract from community providers, the problem with POSHs is the problem of all market reform—a broad array of health care values will be replaced by a narrow set of economic values.

Specialty hospitals deliver the most profitable health care services: cardiac, orthopedic, and general surgical care. To date, market reformers' hopes that physicians will invest in centers for holistic chronic disease management have not materialized. Meeting the broader obligations for community care depends on balancing a range of health priorities and redirecting funding streams as needed. Such ethical decisions have been made in large part by community hospitals. The shift of planning authority toward physician entrepreneurs reconfigures the multiple centers of authority that held sway in community hospitals, where administrators balanced different physician interests over against each other and with community concerns. Such balance is threatened by specialist owners who may not have the full needs of the community in mind as they diligently apply themselves to their area of expertise and the treatment of their patients. As physicians create discrete delivery structures, the result is a partial vision of good health care without any formal structure for opening up that vision to a community's overall needs and the competing values that must be balanced.

Market reformers' claims that physician ownership will usher in an era of transparency are belied by the narrow values that POSHs serve. A director of spiritual care at a large Catholic system questioned how transparent they really are. Even if some POSHs offer "very efficient, cost-effective, high quality care," he asks what gets left out of their facility's ratings. No disclosure is made if "they don't take the really sick people here [but] send them to [the] competitor and skew their mortality rates downward."[29] "That doesn't get published to the consumer. So it's really not a full disclosure. The transparency's a partial transparency."[30]

The work of a Jewish hospital on racial disparities in breast cancer survival rates offers an instructive contrast. An epidemiological research center joined to this hospital discovered a twenty-point gap in survival rates for white and black women in its urban area. One culprit was screening protocols that contributed to an under-diagnosis of breast cancer in African American women, and the hospital advocated a citywide adoption of new radiology standards and a full review of every hospital's performance. In taking the lead, the hospital publicized its screening rates despite shortfalls in its performance. In the words of the hospital's chief executive officer, "Now, we didn't have the best [results]. We had some weaknesses in our own numbers. But we felt it was important enough to raise the issue and be transparent enough to share that publicly. So we partnered with another hospital that had a pretty active breast cancer program and went public."

Here is an example of full transparency answering to an array of values. It began with a commitment to equity in using the hospital's resources to discover a disparity that tracked along racial lines. It continued with a commitment to excellence in hunting down problems that normally would not show in patient outcomes because ratings focus on the treatment stage, not the screening stage. It proceeded with a commitment to integrity in disclosing the hospital's inadequate performance to draw attention to the problem. It culminated in a commitment to community accountability in the creation of a task force to study and improve care across the city. As a consequence, earlier detection for African American women should lead to better health outcomes for them and less costly treatments too. This approach models a fully social transparency through mission-driven structures.

Social transparency and market transparency are not the same. Market transparency stops short at the cost and quality measures of competitors. But efficient use of health care resources is not simply a question of how many procedures at what cost a single facility has performed. A fuller gauge of efficiency must factor in the social costs generated by delayed care when evaluations are not performed, or not performed well, by hospitals overburdened with emergency and charity care. Likewise, quality in health care cannot be equated with a single facility's health outcomes, particularly if those ratings are propped up by sending the hard cases to another hospital, erasing the negatives in the community's health from the positives in one's outcomes data. In short, quality ratings must account for the persistent inequities and inadequacies in community health.

Social transparency does not stop at the cost and quality measures that an organization publishes to grow its market share. Instead, it assesses cost and quality from the standpoint of community care. At the physician level, social transparency would require physicians with privileges at multiple hospitals to publish their quality ratings from their specialty hospital and community hospital locations together. At the hospital level, it would adjust a hospital's quality ratings based on the severity of its cases and its patients' risk factors. At the community level, it would identify shortfalls in care to detect and prevent these deficiencies. Such measures will not create structures of solidarity on their own, but they will point to gaps where people with adequate insurance and secure access do not share in other people's risks, costs, and hardships. The remedies will require coordinated action by committed organizations working in partnership rather than narrowly competing for market share.

The need for transparency measures that answer to a broader array of values can be seen in another health care market, the competition for capital investment. The explosion in capital expenditures is clearest in the race to the suburbs after privately insured patients. In this race safety-net hospitals suffer doubly. Their weak balance sheets force them to pay higher interest rates on loans. Their facilities are often so deteriorated that they can figure little depreciation into their cost basis, reducing their reimbursement levels from government payers. Without access to capital, their ability to compete for privately insured patients worsens, cementing their position as providers of last resort. Disproportionate share hospital payments (see chapter 3) assist with operating costs but not capital expenditures. Nor do federal guarantees of these hospitals' bond ratings put them on a footing to compete for paying patients. Most health care consumers only see the new equipment and shiny facilities at expanding hospital systems, not the increasing financial and geographic distances in health care. Nor do they see the policy structures meant to cushion disparities, operating far out of view.

Although price and quality transparency are both vital, there must also be a broader commitment to making the unfair privileges and burdens in US health care transparent, too. A proposal by the Jewish safety-net hospital CEO helps link the competitive forces operating in the capital market to the social consequences of the hospital race to the suburbs. In the name of *tzedakah*, the covenanted duty to provide financial assistance to the poor, he allowed that his competitors "can have that strong bottom line out [in the suburbs], but [they] also have an obligation to support the rest of the community in some way, whether they tithe in the legal term, whether they get taxed, or they have to set up a foundation to support it." This straightforward appeal to tzedakah is likely to fall on deaf ears, however, because religious values apart from structures mean little in health care. The call to tithe or to create a foundation requires deep structures of solidarity. Yet market reforms are eroding the structures of solidarity that have operated in US health care. This loss of solidarity will frustrate the goal of quality care delivered efficiently and fairly. In today's shifting health care market, shoring up the hidden structures of solidarity and publicizing the pressing need for renewed solidarity are among the most important contributions that religious providers can make toward reform.

STRUCTURING SOLIDARITY INTO US HEALTH CARE

Solidarity is not a value that trips easily off the tongues of many Americans. In American political culture, solidarity means socialism. Solidarity puts taxpayers on the hook for other people's irresponsibility. By shielding consumers from their personal health expenditures, solidarity removes the salutary effects of market choice in disciplining cost and rewarding innovation. In rejecting the notion that health care is a public good, market reformers seek to unleash consumer purchasing power and provider profits to drive decisions about what health care commodities are produced and how they are delivered. Standing in the way are the hidden structures of solidarity that have operated in US health care: the relatively high insurance premiums paid by young and healthy people, the larger share of health care costs borne by big firms, the shifting of uncompensated care losses onto private insurers, and the redirection of hospital revenues from profit centers like cardiac care to money losers like psychiatric care. Note, however, that these structures operate independently of government oversight. They are social structures not public programs, which is why I prefer the more encompassing language of social good over public good.

In calling for personal responsibility, consumer empowerment, and physician innovation, market reformers aim to cut costs and improve quality by giving more control to patients and physicians. They also seek much-needed transparency. These goals are worthy, but market means are insufficient to the task in the absence of a basic solidarity.

Two words capture the problem: market segmentation. The scale and complexity of US health care make it too easy to segment markets by patient risk, geographic location, service line, and insurance coverage. If consumer purchasing power drives decisions about how to structure health coverage and health care, then insurers and providers will slice out the most profitable policyholders from the general population and the most profitable services and locations in US health care. Once segmented, a feedback loop is likely to emerge as market success breeds market success. The insurance company that offers HDHPs chosen by the young and the healthy will see its risks fall, profits rise, and costs drop, pulling even more young and healthy policyholders out of other riskier, more expensive insurance pools. The physician who treats the relatively healthy and wealthy will have the excellent health outcomes to attract better-informed and likely more affluent consumers. The specialty hospital without an emergency department will reduce costs by excluding uninsured patients, allowing the surgeon owners to tout their apparent efficiency in delivering more cost-effective care on a per-patient basis. The profitable organization will gain superior access to cheaper capital for future investments. Consumers with access to these locations will benefit from the lower cost and higher quality, in part by freeing themselves from the solidarity surcharges they have so far paid without their knowledge. Yet purchasing economy for some consumers at the expense of solidarity with sicker, older, and less affluent Americans will generate more in social costs for taxpayers than it yields in consumer gains.

In theory, chronic disease management of diabetes, heart disease, high blood pressure, and other conditions that disproportionately affect poor populations could become a profit center in US health care given the abundant and growing need.[31] In this scenario, better economy and better care could reach people who have not benefited from market reform, and these worthy values would be served by market forces not conscious solidarity. But how can poor Americans pay even the reduced cost of holistic chronic care with a consumer-directed health plan that they must fund on their own? At the very least, the minimal solidarity of public vouchers for insurance plans and public contributions to health savings accounts is prerequisite to this supposedly "market-driven" reform. The public good aspects of health care are very hard to separate from its commodity side. More importantly, the fact that physician entrepreneurs have not invested in chronic disease centers in low-income neighborhoods suggests that this kind of market segmentation by *high* patient risk and *low* patient resource is unlikely even with taxpayers subsidizing HDHPs.

The regional CEO quoted in the epigraph to this chapter sketched out a six-part reform plan at odds with his former free-market beliefs. Because "health care is a public good and a scarce commodity," he proposed structuring US health care as a utility. Without developing the details, an outline shows that solidarity is an operative value throughout his vision, which includes (1) community rating of all insurance policies (policyholders pay the same premiums regardless of their health risks), (2) play-or-pay mandate for all employers (employers who do not provide employee coverage must pay into a general fund for uncovered Americans), (3) universal access insurance (one national insurance pool covers all Americans who have no other insurance), (4) utility commissions set fair rates to pay physicians, pharmacies, pharmaceutical and medical device manufacturers, hospitals, and other health care companies, (5) nonprofit providers lose their tax exemptions for providing uncompensated care, and (6) a strict certificate of need program, insulated from all political influence, determines capital investments in new construction and technology. The CEO observed that his plan may seem "draconian," but he argued that these structures of solidarity are all essential to successful reform.

The 2006 Massachusetts health care reform, which was the model for the ACA, differs from both this utility plan and pure market reform. We see its balance of market mechanisms and structures of solidarity in two key components. First, it created a new health insurance exchange, the Health Connector, through which private insurers offer group policies to residents who were formerly on their own in the expensive individual insurance markets. The goal of the exchange is to build solidarity into the former high-risk, high-cost markets without relying on a public health plan. Second, the law's individual mandate required residents without either employer-sponsored insurance or public insurance to purchase a private insurance policy. This mandate built on the existing structures of solidarity in Massachusetts' regulation of the private insurance industry. Previous reforms had established modified community rating, required guaranteed issue and renewal, and restricted denials for preexisting conditions. As a health policy analyst observed, without these protections, "you have no moral basis to even consider mandating that people have to buy into that kind of a rigged [insurance] market." Everyone's buying in together is what the Massachusetts mandate requires—literally.

The next chapter examines the Massachusetts reform as a basis for the design of the 2010 Affordable Care Act. It also describes how religious activists built solidarity behind implementation of the Massachusetts law. A comment by health policy expert Lawrence Brown on the failed Clinton reform in the 1990s remains pertinent. Even after the ACA, health care reform is stymied by "missing moral momentum." Brown cautions against interpreting some Americans' resistance to government-mandated universal coverage as a moral failing. In his words, people "who are convinced that affordable universal coverage is a moral imperative" should not assume that "those who wish to think twice about it are ethically challenged." Instead Brown calls for conversations in union halls, civic clubs, and religious congregations where people can educate themselves about the complexities of health care and safely explore the values in arguments for different paths toward reform.[32]

Religious health care organizations must contribute to these conversations by bringing their articulated values to the health care reform debate. They can begin by demonstrating where their mission integration responds to the problems of market segmentation. Consider how this might happen if these organizations made their own delivery structures more transparent. I asked a marketing official at a Catholic system how their value of "service of the poor" applied to a flashy billboard campaign I saw while driving along a nearby highway. Her answer was candid: "The market research shows . . . if I were to market the same way [the local safety-net hospital] does, I'd make them my competition versus the teaching institution." Yet if marketing is limited to high-profile services for well-positioned consumers, how is the public to know about this Catholic organization's outreach through the community centers it funds, its community needs assessment, and its subsidized services? If these commitments are touted only in the annual community benefits report because privately insured patients will take their business elsewhere if confronted with other people's access struggles, then the public's understanding of US health care will remain dangerously distorted. This hospital should add a billboard celebrating its charity care initiatives and encouraging the public to join in solidarity.[33]

Clearly there are risks in publicizing mission-driven efforts to improve health care in a competitive environment. Where market share is jealously guarded, the temptation will be great to pursue the values of economy and solidarity in different ways at different times. But who will connect the dots between the values of economy and solidarity if religious health care nonprofits do not take the lead? They have built structures balancing a range of economic and communal values, and they need to bring all of their values to the public debate. As Jewish ethicist Elliot Dorff has noted, the soaring costs of health care make us all potentially poor but may also inspire a new sense of solidarity as more middle-class people are priced out of health insurance or face medical bankruptcy.[34] Religious providers can build on this incipient solidarity, taking the risk of communicating their whole structures, the entire body of their community care initiatives. They should also publicize the unmet needs and priorities that lie beyond their reach due to their own financial limitations or to entrenched structural injustices in the financing and delivery of health care. Given Americans' assumptions about the "private" nature of US health care, it is not surprising that religious providers act as if they must keep economy and solidarity at arm's length. If they try to clap with one hand at a time, however, then the reform debate will once again lack the articulated values needed to generate the moral momentum for meaningful and lasting reform.

NOTES

1. Catholic Health Association, "Fast Facts," www.chausa.org/Pages/Newsroom/Fast_Facts/ (accessed Apr. 10, 2012).

2. Carlson and Galloro, "Big Dividends."

3. See Kleinke, "The Conservative Case for Obamacare."

4. In the early 1990s, hospital occupancy rates hovered around 50 percent, with costs breaking down as follows: 54 percent for labor costs, 37 percent for nonlabor costs, and 9 percent for capital costs (Barr, *Introduction to U.S. Health Policy*, 91).

5. "Hospitals now count on Medicaid for 17 percent of total revenue—almost twice as much as they did two decades ago" (Quinn, "New Directions," 269).

6. Herzlinger, "Why We Need Consumer-Driven Health Care," 105–7. For a critical assessment of POSH as "focused factories," see Casalino et al., "Focused Factories."

7. Kaiser Family Foundation, "Exhibit 6.8," *Employer Health Benefits 2012*.

8. Kaiser Family Foundation, "Exhibit 5.1," *Employer Health Benefits 2012*.

9. Data for 2006 from Medicare Payment Advisory Commission, *Physician-Owned Specialty Hospitals Revisited*. Data for 2010 from Perry, "Physician-Owned Specialty Hospitals," 401. The Physician Hospitals of America, a trade group, identified 277 physician-owned hospitals in 2012 (Robeznieks, "Fight and Flight").

10. Bazzoli et al., "Trends: Construction Activity in U.S. Hospitals."

11. The 1996 Health Insurance Portability and Accountability Act piloted tax-deferred Medical Savings Accounts paired with high-deductible health plans. The 2003 Medicare Prescription Drug, Improvement and Modernization Act replaced them with tax-free Health Savings Accounts for individuals and tax-free Health Reimbursement Accounts funded by employers and employees.

12. Herzlinger, *Consumer-Driven Health Care*, xxii, xxiv.

13. McDonough, *Can a Health Care Market Be Moral?*, 56–57.

14. For an interesting discussion of the multiple effects of commodifying health care, see Kaveny, "Commodifying the Polyvalent Good of Health Care."

15. Roob and Verma, "Indiana: Health Care Reform amidst Clashing Values."

16. The RAND Health Insurance Experiment found evidence that low-income patients with high deductibles decreased their preventive and necessary care. See Gruber, "The Role of Consumer Copayments for Health Care," 5–6.

17. The lack of transparent pricing—let alone consistent pricing—in U.S. health care is vividly detailed in Brill, "Bitter Pill."

18. Cahill, *Theological Bioethics*, 239–40.

19. For arguments that price discrimination, not cost shifting, is the real issue in U.S. health care, see Frakt, "How Much Do Hospitals Cost Shift?"

20. Rosenthal and Daniels, "Beyond Competition," 678–82.

21. Some religious health systems have tried to limit structured dissent by opposing unions. An ethics director in a Catholic system reported having to tell his human resource department that "in our tradition when workers organize they don't become aliens. They're still our employees, they just happen now to be organized." Only where dissent is fully structured can mission and values be fully shared.

22. For Elshtain, placing psychiatrists in primary care clinics would be akin to tracking down the "dysfunctional" who "do not yet know it" to bring them "to wellness" ("Health Care Reform and Finitude," 67).

23. In the Medicare Prescription Drug, Improvement and Modernization Act of 2003, specialty hospitals are defined as "primarily or exclusively engaged in the care and treatment of one of the following categories: (i) patients with a cardiac condition, (ii) patients with an orthopedic condition, and (iii) patients receiving a surgical procedure" (Greenwald et al., "Specialty Versus Community Hospitals," 107).

24. Herzlinger, *Market-Driven Health Care*, 179–81.

25. Greenwald, "Specialty Versus Community Hospitals," 112, 117.

26. Guterman, "Specialty Hospitals," 100.

27. A less rosy study found that physician-owned specialty hospitals and community hospitals had equivalent health outcomes for cardiac revascularization surgery, despite the fact that POSHs treated the relatively healthy and wealthy (Cram et al., "Cardiac Revascularization in Specialty and General Hospitals").

28. Perry, "Physician-Owned Specialty Hospitals," 401–4.

29. A 2006 study commissioned by the Centers for Medicare and Medicaid Services found that physician owners were likelier to treat a healthier population at their facilities than at community hospitals. Medicare Payment Advisory Commission, *Physician-Owned Specialty Hospitals Revisited*, v.

30. In the words of medical ethicist Larry Churchill, "To draw a line around one's actions with the selected group of patients one happens to see personally is to succumb

to precisely the sort of individualist morality that has sustained the inequities in health care for so long" (*Rationing Health Care in America*, 109).

31. According to the Centers for Disease Control, treatments of noncommunicable, preventable chronic diseases constitute 75 percent of U.S. health care costs ("Chronic Diseases", 2).

32. Brown, "Health Reform in America," 103, 111.

33. Cochran cites the need for sacramentality in Catholic health care that unites ministry and advocacy ("Institutional Identity," 35–36).

34. Dorff, *Matters of Life and Death*, 307.

Chapter 6

Building Solidarity
RELIGIOUS ACTIVISM AND SOCIAL JUSTICE

> People in all walks, all across the state [of Massachusetts], everyone understood the problem, and it was really trying to figure out solutions that we could all live with, and that's what health care reform is. It's that solution that puts us all at the table and keeps us all at the table. There are certainly things that we don't like about the reform plan, but there are certainly things that the industry doesn't like about it. There are things that the state doesn't like about it. So we're compromising, making sure that it's statewide, that it's sustainable—not just going to fall away with the next administration.
>
> Volunteer organizer, Greater Boston Interfaith Organization

WHILE CONGRESSIONAL DEMOCRATS were drafting health care reform legislation in 2009, the Tea Party movement emerged as a force in American politics. The Affordable Care Act and the Tea Party can be thought of as fratricidal twins. They grew up together, and the antipathy between their supporters mimics an intense sibling rivalry. The conflict is over Americans' values and their role in reforming US health care. Tea Partiers insist that every American exercise personal responsibility in driving health care toward market efficiency. Supporters of the ACA charge Americans with a shared responsibility for making health care a common good.

As the Affordable Care Act moves into full implementation, it faces a serious legitimacy problem. The Tea Party movement symbolizes cultural resistance to the law. Political resistance can be seen in many states' decision not to set up their own health insurance exchange or expand their Medicaid program. At the core of this resistance are the complementary values of personal liberty and personal responsibility. The prominence of these values in American culture creates an ideal echo chamber for the two main arguments against the ACA: It creates harmful new entitlements, and it wastes taxpayer money.

To date, liberals' counterarguments have not been persuasive. They have relied on the established repertoire of arguments for a right to universal coverage and its economic benefits. On the one hand, liberals have argued that universal coverage is not an entitlement but rather a precondition for the fair equality of opportunity needed to exercise personal liberty. This argument is easily tripped up, however, by the rejoinder that, if personal liberty is the goal, then liberty should not be infringed by higher taxes or by mandates to buy health insurance. On the other hand, liberals cite the economic savings to be found in universal coverage of preventive, primary, and chronic care versus the expense of deferred care and emergency care. This economic argument runs afoul, however, of the belief that private enterprise and consumer choice are always more efficient than government regulation.

Tea Party opposition to the ACA has gone well beyond appeals to personal liberty and personal responsibility in rejecting mainstream liberal and economic arguments. The grassroots movement has also drawn on iconic images of the Boston Tea Party and laid claim to the rights language and antitax protests that provoked revolution against British colonialism. Compared to the Tea Party's embrace of the historical legacy of revolutionary liberty, the defense of the ACA by its supporters has been tepid, technical, and, not surprisingly, unpersuasive to roughly half of Americans.[1]

This chapter examines another activist group, the Greater Boston Interfaith Organization (GBIO), a coalition of Christian, Jewish, and now Muslim congregations along with union locals, civic groups, and community development centers. The organization participated in the Affordable Care Today! (ACT) coalition that championed the 2006 Massachusetts health care reform law. GBIO delivered people to the cause by collecting 100,000 petition signatures, staging regular demonstrations at the Massachusetts State House, and connecting journalists to uninsured people living outside the usual media spotlight. Although much smaller than the Tea Party movement, GBIO claimed its own historical legacy—the idea of the Commonwealth of Massachusetts as a city on a hill and founding covenant of American community. They also created a public liturgy of health care reform that injected religious values into the Massachusetts debate. In so doing, GBIO fostered solidarity among people inside and outside the organization.

Solidarity in health care means a conscious willingness to sacrifice financially and set shared priorities to ensure an inclusive, fair, efficient, and sustainable system.[2] Solidarity is a collective determination to stand with others, asking whether one could live with their health care options. It calls for community action to reorganize health care delivery toward prevention, wellness, and cost-effective care, even when those changes require accepting limits on personal care options. In the words of a GBIO activist, health care reform is "that solution that puts us all at the table and keeps us all at the table." Solidarity is the missing element in the ACA's cultural and political legitimacy. It is the missing backdrop to secular liberal and economic arguments for universal coverage. The ACA will not succeed without a solidarity supplement from a "We Party" movement that strikes covenantal chords of everyone's being at the table—both in having covered access to health care and in taking responsibility for paying into and managing the cost of the system. The future direction of health care reform depends on whether Americans can make solidarity a cornerstone value of US health care. If not, the ACA will likely sputter and flame out, ushering in an era of market-driven reform.

Understanding how GBIO activists brought their religious values into the public sphere advances two theses of this book. First, US health care operates as a social good much more than Americans recognize. The social good of US health care has been built up through public investments in such values as innovation, fairness, compassion, and equity (chapter 3). It has been extended through community benefits policy (chapter 4) and structured into religious nonprofits' delivery of health care (chapter 5). Nevertheless, public recognition about how much US health care already operates as a social good is not widespread.

Second, religious values can strengthen Americans' commitment to making health care a more complete social good. The two previous chapters described how religious nonprofits aspire to provide community benefits based on the moral ideals of covenant and common good and how they strive to give concrete meaning to their mission and values in their operational and delivery structures. This chapter takes the next step—from moral ideals to articulated values to public norms. GBIO's interfaith activism engaged its members' convictions, leading them to enact their Jewish and Christian values as shared values inside the organization and to communicate them to the broader public. Activists worked out quasi-public understandings of religious values that were taken into the political debate over the state's policies. The success of GBIO demonstrates how important religious congregations, interfaith coalitions, and religious health care nonprofits can be to the national debate.

CHAPTER 58: ACHIEVEMENTS
AND LIMITATIONS

Massachusetts' health care reform law, known as Chapter 58, is the model for the ACA. In Massachusetts, however, the legislation was drafted and passed with bipartisan cooperation. In starting the process, Republican governor Mitt Romney insisted that any reform plan include an individual mandate that residents obtain health coverage from an employer, a public program, or a new state insurance exchange of private health plans called the Health Connector. Residents who failed to meet the mandate were subject to fines up to the value of their state personal tax exemption. Democrats countered that if coverage was mandated, then public subsidies were needed to help residents earning up to 300 percent of the federal poverty level (FPL) afford it.

A bipartisan compromise created a three-tiered structure of coverage for people without insurance through an employer or Medicare. First, MassHealth, the state's Medicaid program, was expanded to cover all children living in families below 300 percent of FPL and all adults earning less than 150 percent of FPL. Second, the new Commonwealth Care plans for adults earning between 150 and 300 percent of FPL were subsidized on a sliding scale by income. Finally, the Health Connector offered the new Commonwealth Choice plans to people earning over 300 percent of FPL. Although the Choice plans are unsubsidized, they cost less than equivalent private individual policies because the insurance exchange pools policyholders into larger risk groups. Special discount policies were also offered to young adults. By comparison, the ACA guarantees Medicaid coverage up to 133 percent of FPL (unless a state adopts a higher level or chooses not to participate). The ACA's subsidies for policies purchased through state insurance exchanges slide up to 400 percent of FPL.

In contrast to the bitter partisan divides over the ACA, Chapter 58 passed with only two dissenting votes out of the 193 votes cast. This near unanimity reflected the broad acceptance of two principles at the heart of the bill. First, there would be "shared responsibility" for the cost of expanded coverage. Shared sacrifice was required by all of the major stakeholders, including businesses, insurers, providers, government, and consumers. Businesses with more than ten employees were subject to a "fair share contribution" of $295 per employee if they did not cover at least 25 percent of their full-time employees or pay at least 33 percent of their full-time employees' premiums. Insurers lost the profitable individual insurance market. Hospitals and physicians gained higher reimbursements for their MassHealth patients, but hospitals and health centers began losing state safety-net funding. The state's health care budget increased significantly to pay for the Medicaid expansion and the Commonwealth Care subsidies. Finally, some consumers contributed more to the system through the individual mandate or tax penalties for failing to abide by it.

These five stakeholder groups were also represented on the Health Connector board, an oversight board charged with defining the law's second principle:

residents can only be mandated to purchase "creditable, affordable coverage." Creditable coverage establishes the baseline of services that must be included in policies sold on the insurance exchange. Affordable coverage caps the premiums that residents at different income levels can be expected to pay. Simply put, the principle of "creditable, affordable coverage" establishes the claims and limits of solidarity in a health care system that includes nearly all residents. By handing this issue to the Health Connector board, the Massachusetts legislature avoided a fractious legislative debate. More importantly, it instigated a public conversation about the meaning of shared responsibility in health care. GBIO and its allies weighed in, successfully lobbying for a more forgiving process of waiving fines on residents who are financially unable to purchase creditable, affordable coverage.

Chapter 58's achievements have been considerable. In 2010 (the most recent data available), estimates of health coverage in Massachusetts ranged from a high of 98 percent of residents to a low of 96 percent, compared to 84 percent for the nation.[3] During the law's first four years, coverage rates for nonelderly adults rose from 87 percent to 94 percent (compared to 78 percent for the United States).[4] In addition, the law has accomplished the following:

1. improved patients' access and continuity of care (though "unmet need" rose 3 percent from 2009 to 2010 because of the recession)[5]
2. increased the percentage of firms offering health insurance from 70 percent in 2005 to 77 percent in 2010, contrary to predictions that Chapter 58 would lead employers to dump coverage onto the state[6]
3. reduced public spending on uncompensated care from $652 million (fiscal year 2006) to $414 million (fiscal year 2009)[7]
4. decreased patient visits to emergency departments, even as emergency visits increased nationally[8]
5. held annual inflation in the Commonwealth Care program below 2 percent per enrollee.[9]

These accomplishments explain why support for the law remains steady at nearly two-thirds of Massachusetts residents (65.6 percent in 2010), even as unfavorable views of the law have also increased, rising from 17 to 27 percent since the law's passage.[10]

The chief shortcoming of Chapter 58 has been its inability to halt rising health care costs. Massachusetts has the highest per capita health care spending in the United States, and its growth trend continued through the first two years of the new law.[11] Cost increases were not surprising, however, given Chapter

58's primary goal of expanding creditable, affordable health coverage. Now that the principle of shared responsibility has taken hold and more patients are walking in the front door of the health care system, legislators have shifted their attention to controlling costs. In August 2012, Gov. Deval Patrick signed a bill that, among other provisions, pegs annual growth in health care spending to annual growth in the state's economy.

The high cost of health care is a principal complaint against Chapter 58 on both the right and the left. Tom Miller, a health economist at the American Enterprise Institute, offers a view from the right: "Massachusetts is a very high-cost state for health care, with a concentrated market of relatively inefficient providers already swimming in a sea of dysfunctional public subsidies and crippling overregulation."[12] From the perspective of market reform, increasing public subsidies to an already expensive health industry and authorizing an oversight board to define creditable and affordable coverage precludes the market discipline and personal liberty of consumer choice.

From the political left, advocates of a single-payer system argue that only a government-run health plan can guarantee cost control and universal coverage. A hybrid system of public mandates for private health policies does not eliminate the administrative overhead and profits of private insurers. Requiring uninsured residents to purchase private insurance or be fined was seen as a huge step backward by single-payer liberals.[13] GBIO also had grave concerns about the individual mandate. As described by a rabbi on their leadership team, GBIO swallowed

> this very, very bad-tasting medicine on the condition that it would mean more people will get access and that nobody would get punished who can't afford it. We won that. What we didn't win, which we never thought we were going to win, is universal coverage. But you've had all the people on the extreme who have been sitting in the wilderness on their own holding up signs saying that it's [the single-payer] way or no way, and then nothing happened. Tell [GBIO member] Peter Brooke we should hold out for universal health care. Peter Brooke now has an affordable health plan that he did not have a year ago.

As we shall see, GBIO not only reluctantly accepted the individual mandate as a political compromise, they ultimately embraced it as the moral linchpin of a socially just American health care system committed to the principles of shared responsibility, creditable care, and affordable coverage.

RELIGIOUS ACTIVISM AND
PARTICIPANT VALUES

This overview of Chapter 58 sets the stage for understanding GBIO's contributions to the Massachusetts debate, from lobbying for its passage through advocating for its full implementation. As a congregation-based community organizer, GBIO engages in community activism and public advocacy in response to members' concerns and commitments. The resulting dynamic between social action and public argument channels the experiential knowledge gained in a community of conviction into a shared participant language. A comparison with the Tea Party movement is instructive. Although more about political protest than community organizing, Tea Partiers created political rituals that acted out a narrative of revolutionary liberty to induce other Americans to feel the emotional hold and renewed practical relevance of an iconic symbol of American values. Whether a grassroots movement is secular or religious, conservative or liberal, it can generate a distinctive public language, the power of which flows from the states of moral conviction and emotional uplift that activists attain on their journey together.

Catholic ethicist Lisa Sowle Cahill coined the phrase "participatory discourse" to account for the formative dynamic that can transpire between participant activism and moral language. When activist groups engage their base, conduct their meetings, serve their communities, protest public policies, and so forth, they express and exercise their moral commitments together, giving concrete shape and living presence to their values. As an illustration, consider the public argument offered by GBIO president and senior pastor of Roxbury Presbyterian Church, Rev. Hurmon Hamilton, in a June 2007 post on radio station WBUR's *CommonHealth* blog. In a title echoing throughout his post, Hamilton appealed to scripture declaring, "This is the day the LORD has made; let us rejoice and be glad in it (Psalms 118:24, New International Version)."[14] The cause for celebration was the life-affirming experiences of newly insured GBIO members. Rejoicing at every turn, Hamilton recounted the benefits for Peter Brooke, a construction worker with untreated diabetes; for Kristin Bonelli, a recent college graduate working two part-time jobs; and for Lavern Barnes, a woman in her mid-fifties whose first covered trip to a doctor revealed a life-threatening condition, for which she now had insurance to cover the treatment. In Hamilton's closing words: "Surely this is the day that the LORD has made, let us rejoice and be glad in it!"[15] Hamilton's public sermonizing advanced and defined the public norm of protecting life. As with other religious ethics of life, this one presupposes a list of divine commandments—preventing early morbidity, avoiding financial disaster, averting treatable fatal conditions, and sharing responsibility for meeting the social costs of these duties.

When an activist group brings their participant values to public debates, their arguments may not conform to the secular principles and neutral policy terms demanded by many liberals. Instead, as Cahill observes, the language's "persuasive value derives only in part from its intellectual coherence. It derives in equal measure from its power to allude to or induce a shared sphere of behavior, oriented by shared concerns and goals, and its power to constitute relations of empathy and interdependence among the 'arguers.'"[16] This dynamic linkage among shared actions, shared concerns, and shared goals defines GBIO's work to nurture relationships within member congregations and to draw these congregations into wider interfaith cooperation.

Building "relational power" is how the rabbi on GBIO's leadership team described the process of cultivating empathy and interdependence. During our interview, I naively asked if his affluent synagogue had supported the health care reform campaign out of a sense of social despair that so many other Americans were uninsured. The rabbi rejected this "we/they" thinking as hopelessly distant: "In my experience people rarely stand in the rain to collect signatures out of some abstract sense of social despair." Instead, members of his temple became personally invested by joining small house meetings where their fellow Jews told their health care stories. At every meeting, the rabbi found, even if participants "didn't have their own personal narrative [of financial struggles or access problems], they were in a relational network" with someone who did. Thus the synagogue's desire to work for health care reform was first made intimate and then expansive through the house meetings.

A lay Congregationalist member reported how working with GBIO helped renew her stultifyingly intellectual church. Congregants were challenged to become more expressive about their faith, making them accountable "to whatever faith we bring to the table. We're accountable to each other, and we're accountable to our peers." Empathy can breathe life into what were once only intellectual commitments to the moral obligations of one's tradition. Interdependence across an interfaith coalition can translate religious convictions into community action and advocacy for public policies.

Although the experiential and relational content of an activist group's participant values may seem to preclude outsiders' reasoned understanding, Cahill identifies a strategy for public communication: "Effectiveness requires both the deployment of a vocabulary and imagery with broad cultural appeals and the cultivation of grassroots practices and communities that display and reinforce that imagery."[17] In other words, bridging the gap between participant values and public deliberation requires well-chosen words and images that invite outsiders into familiar and habitable imaginative spaces embodying the purpose and power of insiders' social actions and moral attitudes. Hamilton's *CommonHealth* posts tell the outer tale of GBIO's participant values. Two representative actions highlight the genesis of these public arguments in members' grassroots actions and relationship building.

One of GBIO's most consequential actions was holding seventy affordability workshops at which six hundred participants tallied up their incomes and expenses to discern how much they could afford in health expenditures under the individual mandate. Although not a scientific sample, the collected data became part of the Connector Board's initial deliberation over the state's affordability schedule, which sets the maximum monthly premiums that residents can be expected to pay at different income levels. The lay Congregationalist woman related a transformative experience during one session. Some years before, as a young, educated, self-sufficient adult, she had incurred a huge hospital debt because she did not know that her employer's policy had an annual cap. She was so ashamed by her sense of irresponsibility that she told no one—not her parents, friends, or former employer. Many years passed. Then after being thrust into leading an affordability workshop at a low-income congregation, she told her story for the first time. The congregants had been angry that the subsidies for their mandated coverage were not higher. They demanded to know why the sliding scale of subsidies went to people earning all the way up to 300 percent of FPL. In risking her own story, the GBIO volunteer bridged the empathy gap. Afterward, the group was, in her words, "a bit awestruck; it was transforming for them because they started to understand that even though someone has a higher income, they may be struggling, too; and for me it was transforming just because I said it. I named this thing that I'd been hiding for years from people."

This woman found herself—quite literally—at a table where socioeconomic and racial divisions were overcome through faithful accountability to candid dialogue about health care risk and responsibility. By investing her faith and trust in a group of relative strangers joined with her in a shared action, she experienced the priority of justice over charity in health care reform. In her words, "Charity is something where we keep ourselves distanced from the problem. There's a valley between me, the giver, and the person receiving it. Justice, just in its nature, you have to build that bridge because justice is about saying that your problem is my problem. My problem is your problem. And we're going to fight together to solve that problem, rather than just saying, here's the money, now please go away." In the past her congregation never actually said,

"Here's the money, now please go away." But their previous interfaith donations (e.g., to help rebuild African American churches burned down by arsonists) had the effect of keeping other people's problems at a distance. With GBIO members telling their health care stories in house meetings with fellow congregants, joining with other GBIO congregations in interfaith worship services, and continuing into shared actions like the affordability workshops, a growing empathy and sense of common purpose made room for participants to take personal risks and adjust assumptions about other people's realities. Entrenched economic myths and social divisions were unsettled, and a new space of solidarity shifted religious commitments from the minimal aid of charity to the fulsome response of justice. Built over the course of many actions, the solidarity among GBIO members forged an empathetic interdependence and gave priority to social justice over distant charity.

These commitments to solidarity and social justice were not confined inside GBIO. The members extended their participant values through door-to-door canvassing to teach residents about the individual mandate and their coverage options. These participant values flowed into Hamilton's *CommonHealth* posts, nearly all of which opened with a scriptural epigraph or title. One of his posts opened with the story of Jesus's words to a man who for thirty-eight years had been lying paralyzed by the pool of Bethesda: "When Jesus saw him and knew he had been ill for a long time, he asked him, 'Would you like to get well?' 'I can't, sir,' the sick man said, 'for I have no one to put me into the pool when the water bubbles up. Someone else always gets there ahead of me.' Jesus told him, 'Stand up, pick up your mat, and walk!' Instantly the man was healed! (John 5:6–9, New Living Translation)." Applying this verse to the "wonder" of Chapter 58 on the second anniversary of its passage, Hamilton explained that once a year an angel would stir up bubbles in the pool, offering a miracle of healing to the first person into the waters. The analogy is to charity care. The lines of people waiting in emergency departments for the handout of charity care had been replaced for over 340,000 Massachusetts residents by the time of this post. Standing up, walking to an enrollment center, and taking one's place in the health care system is more than a matter of having secure access. It takes moral growth for people accustomed to economic queuing for care that is already rationed for uninsured and underinsured people. Moral growth is required by others, too, Hamilton continued. Jesus's compassion for the sick man is a model for everyone to reach across "language, economic, or other barriers" to enroll residents in coverage. Calling all of the stakeholders in Chapter 58 "angels if you will," Hamilton exhorted them to stir up their own bubbles of systemic change. For uninsured people, that means paying what they can for health coverage. For health care activists, it means continued public pressure. For health care providers, it means cost-effective delivery of care. Everyone's better angel has a contribution to make on the journey to affordable, quality care for all.[18]

This interpretation of the pool of Bethesda story is unusual in two ways. On the one hand, conservative Christian readings highlight the paralytic's purely personal initiative in responding to Jesus's call to health. On this reading Jesus's miraculous powers can heal anyone who stops making excuses about needing other people's assistance and accepts God's forgiveness. Jesus's instruction to the man, "Sin no more, that nothing worse befall you" (John 5:14), locates the cause of his paralysis in the man's faults. Thus, with Christ's forgiving love always available, healing is a personal and spiritual act of faith. GBIO's social actions challenge this spiritualized interpretation of the healing power of inner faith. The pain and struggle encountered in house meetings and neighborhood canvassing call forth a response as neighbor and acknowledge that personal initiative and responsibility are insufficient for people with chronic illness and disability. Carrying out Jesus's healing ministry to body, mind, and soul commands social transformation, including the new insurance structures erected by Chapter 58 and active community outreach by groups like GBIO. Further lessons come from GBIO's interfaith worship. The fifth chapter of the Gospel of John is framed by the conflict between Jesus and Jewish authorities about healing on the Sabbath. In this case it is not social action, but the social presence of GBIO's Jewish members that challenges prejudice. Acknowledging Judaism's longstanding duty of healing even on the Sabbath corrects the supposed pharisaical preference for the letter of the law over the spirit of compassion. Instead, the justice orientation of Jewish ethics makes a purely spiritualized ideal of healing through inner faith grow paler still.

On the other hand, Hamilton's use of this gospel narrative differs from standard liberal arguments for health care reform. His call to the uninsured to stand up and walk to an enrollment center is not simply an appeal for government guarantees of positive rights. His naming all of the stakeholders in Chapter 58 "angels if you will" is more than a poetic linking of a divine calling to a secular social contract. Positive rights and social contracts are the creations of liberal citizens who consent to laws and policies that serve their mutual interests. In the clash of political interests in a liberal democracy, positive rights and social contracts can simply be the accepted rules of fair play. They need not presuppose any unifying vision of the good of health care in a just society. The skeleton of law has to be fleshed out, however, in people's active assent to its legitimacy. In contrast to the ongoing resistance to the ACA, GBIO's actions helped build and inhabit a space of solidarity among citizens. When Hamilton invokes Jesus's charge to "Stand up, pick up your mat, and walk," it summons forth personal initiative and responsibility for oneself and one's fellow citizens, too. The post concludes: "Get up, enroll, and, prayerfully, be healed. And oh by the way, 'we are here to help you!' Happy two year anniversary everybody."[19] Putting the promise of help into action, GBIO canvassers witnessed in the faces of the people they met both the insecurity and isolation caused by lacking insurance and the relief and dignity that affordable, creditable coverage brings. The canvassers experienced compassion, justice, and dignity in action. In relating their stories to fellow GBIO members, the group's participant values were enriched by multiple encounters and new insights into the practical expression of these values.

In all of GBIO's actions—beginning with house meetings and interfaith worship services and continuing into petition drives, visits to elected officials, public protests, and advocacy at agency meetings—values are made concrete, sentiments of solidarity are extended, and the formative moral commitments are re-performed at every retelling of the pool of Bethesda story and the other biblical vignettes in Hamilton's posts.

GBIO'S PUBLIC LITURGY OF
HEALTH CARE REFORM

Participant values are not unique to religious communities, but GBIO's arguments are distinguished by their religious content and form. The content is mostly biblical; the form is liturgical. I use the term liturgy to explain how GBIO's interfaith meetings and Hamilton's posts injected religious values into the Massachusetts debate. A key feature of this liturgical style is its calendrical structure. Over the course of the health care reform campaign, GBIO leaders established a calendar of key dates on the journey from passage through implementation of Chapter 58. Hamilton's blog was the public expression of this liturgy turned into a repeating and building annual cycle. As with any liturgy, however, the significance and interwoven integrity of the expressed values inhere in their performance by the members of a community.

Two different communities are implicit in Hamilton's blog. The first is the community of reform advocates, particularly the Christian and Jewish members of GBIO whose worship in their home congregations and interfaith gatherings was the genesis of the public liturgy. The other community is Massachusetts residents who are all invited to make these religious values their own. In effect,

Hamilton's posts deploy the "public worship" (Latin: *liturgia*) of GBIO members to advance the "public work" (Greek: *leit-ourgos*) of policy change.[20]

The first sense of the term liturgy—public worship—was on display at GBIO's tenth anniversary celebration, an event that drew seventeen hundred GBIO activists and political and corporate leaders. Anticipating the evening's forum, Hamilton's post from earlier that day opened with the epigraph "Come now, and let us reason together (Isaiah 1:18–20, NKJV)." A video of the forum records a lively scene led by Hamilton's scriptural appeals and met by GBIO attendees' call and response: "Send me to write the next chapter"; "Shared power, shared responsibility, shared sacrifice!" With GBIO's relational power swelling and members' values echoing off the walls, Hamilton turned to the assembled legislative and business leaders and exhorted them to solidarity: "Even when we are on different sides of the issues, we will remain at the same table until we find a resolution." To GBIO's members, he pledged, "We will remain at the table with all of our power . . . stay until the job is done, remembering the least of these." Finally, to everyone gathered, he declared, "Surely the spirit of the Lord is upon us tonight!"[21] In the close quarters of this forum, it is easy to see how GBIO's public worship is used to press outsiders into agreement. The policy proposals in Hamilton's posts are offered in the same spirit of joining together as a covenanted community and reasoning on the basis of "common" values, as found in scripture and enacted by GBIO.

These blog posts might well be called policy sermons. Reviewing all nineteen posts, the sense of building liturgical momentum is palpable. Hamilton's first post in February 2007 alludes to Martin Luther King Jr.'s 1967 title *Where Do We Go from Here?*, and there are ecumenical appeals to the preciousness of every human life (Gen. 1:27), the call to act for "the health and wholeness of our community" (Mat. 9:25), and Moses Maimonides's injunction that a "public system of health care is the moral obligation of any just community."[22] Only this first post and the one that followed lack a biblical passage in an epigraph or title, suggesting that Hamilton and his fellow GBIO strategists found their way as they crafted the reform liturgy.

Right from the outset, however, Hamilton combined biblical passages with GBIO's participant values to tell a covenantal story of Chapter 58 and to set the policymaking process within a context of solidarity. His second post on Easter Sunday anticipates the first anniversary of Chapter 58's passage. It exhibits GBIO's philosophy that interfaith strength grows not from diluting religious differences, but from Jews and Christians praying and speaking out of their respective traditions. Hamilton notes the Passover remembrance of the journey

out of slavery, but his title metaphor of "A Dying Hope" is keyed to the resur-
rection. "As I proclaim this morning that Jesus and the hope he embodies is
alive," Hamilton writes, "I am deeply concerned that the hope of health care
reform is being crucified."[23] Moving from biblical story to public policy, he
invokes the religious calendar of his African American Christian tradition to
lend divine significance to a decisive moment in the implementation of Chapter
58. The present threat was the Connector Board's first attempt at setting an
affordability schedule. As already noted, GBIO's affordability data and its activism helped influence the board on this occasion to adopt a more forgiving
schedule than was on the table.

This success elicited Hamilton's first scriptural epigraph in the next post one
month later. His chosen passage rings with the celebration and promise of a
covenant restored. "Enlarge your house; build an addition. Spread out your
home, and spare no expense! For soon you will be bursting at the seams (Isaiah
54:2–3, New Living Translation)." The expectant, almost triumphal tone fit
GBIO's sense of the moment. One year into the law, the Connector Board
had defined creditable and affordable care. The new Commonwealth Care and
Commonwealth Choice plans were ready for enrollees. All of the policy details
were worked out, except for residents and businesses signing on to their responsibilities under the individual and employer mandates. As with any covenantal
ethics, the promise is realized only after everyone makes the necessary sacrifices.
Yet at this moment, Hamilton charges, the funds allocated for outreach and
enrollment had been cut from the state budget. "Spare no expense!" he declares.
"As for us," he imagines the legislators thinking, "the hard work of crafting
reform is finally over [and] we must be spared from the expense of such insig-
nificant activities" as informing residents of the new law and enrolling people
in coverage.[24] For GBIO members, however, action with others marks the start
of defining the values implicit in the reform law and lodging them in the public's
consciousness of moral progress made together.

In addition to addressing the affordability schedule, many of Hamilton's
posts concern Chapter 58's individual mandate. When the individual mandate
came into force in July 2007, his epigraph quoted Jesus's praise for the widow's
mite. "Jesus said, 'I tell you the truth, this poor widow has put more into
the treasury than all the others' (Mark 12:43)." Jesus shows greater respect for
the widow's gift than the large monetary contributions of wealthy benefactors.
The reform value here is the dignity of the poor, not the preferential option for
the poor. Typically supporters of expanded coverage appeal to the needs of
poorer people, not to their financial contributions. But Chapter 58 calls for

shared responsibility, including responsibility exercised by those lower- and middle-income residents mandated to pay into the system. In stepping forward to meet their subsidized or unsubsidized coverage obligations, they contribute to the funding pools that insure everyone, an act of justice performed by 195,000 new policyholders as of June 2009.[25]

In February 2008, Hamilton argued that this commitment to justice by the newly insured must be met by mercy for those residents who are unable to afford their insurance premiums and health care costs. With the Connector Board's annual review of the affordability schedule set for Valentine's Day, his epigraph reads: "Mercy and truth are met together; righteousness and peace have kissed each other (Psalms 85:10)." The willingness of residents to obtain mandated coverage must be joined with forgiveness from undue financial burdens. The post continues as follows: "On the day many people pause to remember promises and re-affirm commitments—the Connector Board members will be presented with an opportunity to remember and re-affirm their promise made last year: the state will not penalize individuals and families in the Commonwealth who cannot afford to purchase the health care—how appropriate."[26] As before, Hamilton clothes the next step in the reform process with a biblical passage, which in this case dovetails with the Valentine's Day celebration of love. The communal message is clear: the spirit of reconciliation and consensus shown thus far must continue. By joining a biblical passage to both the reform calendar and the secular calendar, Hamilton expands GBIO's liturgical efforts to make their participant values public norms. Moral pressure builds on policymakers, too, who are alternately encouraged and chided to heed their promises to act as stewards, not mere financial adjustors, of an evolving equation of mandated contributions and budget overruns.

This collective moral momentum drives the post on the first anniversary of the individual mandate, too. Hamilton asks the meaning of the state's official name, the Commonwealth of Massachusetts. Calling commonwealth the secular equivalent of covenant, he answers, "Simply put, the vision we are called to embrace going forward is 'shared power,' 'shared responsibility,' and 'shared sacrifice.' "[27] If every stakeholder does his or her part in covering *and* containing the costs of expanded access, then affordable, quality health care for all—the new purpose binding the citizens of the commonwealth together—can become a reality.

Heading into summer 2008, new enrollees were increasing the cost of Chapter 58, and recession was threatening. Hamilton warned that health care reform could not stop being the public work of the commonwealth. Quoting Jesus's apocalyptic warning that anyone who neglects to care for "the least of these" will not be reckoned among the righteous (Matthew 25:44–46), Hamilton proclaims that the "character of our Commonwealth" is revealed not in times of surplus, but "during times of scarcity. Who is expendable? Who do we delete from the budget, without a whimper?" He cites the legislature's proposed cut of coverage for the 28,000 legal immigrants in Commonwealth Care.[28] As the financial crisis intensified, another post provided the complementary instruction: "Render to Caesar the things that are Caesar's, and to God the things that are God's (Mark 12:17)." Goodwill alone, Hamilton implies, cannot solve budget problems. Putting the spotlight on businesses, he criticizes the $7 million raised by Chapter 58's supposedly "fair and reasonable" provision for noncovering employers, and he argues that, with uninsured residents stepping forward to pay their portion of new costs, business owners should render a fairer contribution, too.[29]

As the recession took hold the following summer, Hamilton once again challenged the legislature not to cut legal immigrants from subsidized health plans. Addressing the state as one community, he misquotes a familiar passage, "Yea, though [we] walk through the valley of the shadow of death, [we] will fear no evil" (Psalms 23:4, KJV; brackets are Hamilton's). Even in perilous economic times, excluding immigrants who reside legally in Massachusetts is wrong because of (1) the loss of "potentially life-saving preventive and follow-up care," (2) the unfair burden on some of the commonwealth's "most vulnerable and least resourced" residents, (3) the example of retreat when Massachusetts is being considered as a model for national reform, and (4) the capitulation to the federal government's refusal to provide states with matching funds for legal immigrants' care. In Hamilton's words, this federal funding rule is an "evil" threatening the "Soul of our Commonwealth," and noncooperation with evil is the only way to avoid complicity in it.[30]

This sampling of Hamilton's posts conveys how GBIO crafted a liturgy of reform values, drawing on the actions and experiences of its members, sanctifying their struggles and successes with Bible verses, and marking their progress on a calendar of key dates on the journey toward the full promise of Chapter 58. Inspired by the public worship and shared actions of member congregations, this liturgy affirms the values of dignity, justice, mercy, truth, compassion, shared sacrifice, stewardship, civility, and noncomplicity. On this basis, Hamilton argues, health care reform can be a public work of securing the creditable, affordable coverage that the state has mandated for every resident. Raising the needed funds and restraining the escalating costs can succeed only if all of the stakeholders commit to the foundational value of covenantal solidarity.

This solidarity is of a certain kind. It is not unitary and top down; it is experimental and pluralistic. Solidarity emerged from the personal stories, religious appeals, and transforming encounters that took hold in GBIO's worship and actions. The space of moral formation created by these activities is a space opened up by relationship, empathy, and even outrage. In the words of a Catholic organizer, "There's a connection between anger, grief, and empathy. A really skilled rhetorician can help people tap into their empathy through the skillful use of moral outrage." In GBIO's case the moral momentum for health care reform built from the combination of, on the one hand, the community organizing strategies that fueled members' relational power and, on the other hand, a covenantal ethics that channeled this solidarity into a political vision of justice in which affordable, quality health care for all is a public work of the commonwealth and a shared responsibility of every resident. Thus, even as Hamilton urges civility—"Come now, and let us reason together"—GBIO's participant values advance a religious vision of a just society not shared by all Americans. How then should liberal supporters of the ACA view GBIO's socially active and morally tendentious arguments, given secular liberal qualms about religious arguments in public life?

MARKETPLACE JUSTICE OR HEALTH CARE SOLIDARITY

Hamilton's posts address the policy details of Chapter 58 as much as they do the moral lessons of scripture. But GBIO's arguments are not stated in the ostensibly neutral language of public policy—individual rights, state interests, costs, benefits, efficiency, incentives. GBIO's reasoning is framed by stories that speak to the moral growth and empathetic connections behind their participant values. Once abstract and distant, these values have been made vividly alive and practically concrete as GBIO members hammered them out among one other and with the people they helped. Normally, values pull people in a general direction like the polestar leading sailing ships along their independent courses. A construction metaphor is more apt here. By working strategically toward common goals, GBIO activists' trial steps, changes of mind, and growing list of accomplishments brought their values down from the heights of ethereal abstraction. They built their participant values up and out through shared actions and stories, erecting a solid platform of moral commitments and public stances. The more the structure took form, the more it grounded participants' ethical initiative. A Catholic organizer describes GBIO's remarkable combination of integrity and experiment: "We are able to be value driven, but not overly principled. We compromise." Because participant values are experiential and multifaceted, they can be more pragmatically flexible than the principles that intellectuals often bring to the health care reform debate. GBIO's willingness to compromise does not mean, however, that their activism created a neutral space of deliberation. Everyone was called to the policymaking table, but the moral momentum generated by putting religious values into action took some policy options off the table too.

Fundamentally GBIO activists asked, Does health care have to include and serve all of the residents of Massachusetts? If yes, then health care reform must be a matter of solidarity and its governing standard is social justice. If no, then health care reform can answer instead to the meritocratic standard of commutative justice advocated by market reformers and the Tea Party movement.

As developed in chapter 1, commutative justice is also called justice in exchange. This understanding of justice is modeled on voluntary transactions among two or more parties. If the parties exchange goods or services at a mutually agreeable ratio, then their agreement makes for a just exchange, provided that everyone involved has adequate information and no one is manipulated or coerced. Such voluntary transactions of commutative justice contrast with the full participation in community that creates social justice. Catholic ethicist David Hollenbach helpfully breaks social justice into the two categories of contributive justice and distributive justice: "Contributive justice requires that citizens be active members of the community. . . . Distributive justice is, in turn, concerned with the way the members of society share in the goods that life together makes possible."[31] Contributive justice has an outward flow as people's economic risk and labor, social interactions, and cultural dynamism generate a plenitude of goods that become available to other people. Distributive justice has a return flow as the goods we jointly produce are distributed to individuals according to some standard of desert, such as merit, need, effort, or equality. Social justice incorporates and builds upon these two pillars of a just society. It adds the necessity of removing barriers to social participation that leave some citizens unable to contribute to or benefit from the common good.[32]

Distinguishing commutative justice from social justice charts the philosophical poles in the national health care reform debate. At one end, there is commutative justice, the justice of individual choices in the marketplace. At the other end, there is social justice, the commitment to solidarity in health care. Of the two, personal liberty is much more at home in American political culture than is solidarity. As a result, the governing principles of commutative justice—

market choice and individual merit—tend to function as the de facto principles of contributive and distributive justice in the public's mind. By contrast, the ethical pull of covenant and common good is toward shared responsibility and human dignity, moral norms that span Christian and Jewish traditions and even liberal and conservative theologies. Mainstream economic and liberal policy arguments in favor of universal coverage are consonant with the health care values of shared responsibility and human dignity. In the absence of an underlying solidarity in US health care, however, the mechanics of economic efficiency and positive rights struggle to escape from the atomism of justice in exchange and the ideological service it performs for the privileged.[33] GBIO's religious arguments about the ethics of the individual mandate reveal those limitations.

THE ECONOMICS OF THE INDIVIDUAL MANDATE: EFFICIENCY OR SOLIDARITY?

The individual mandate marks the triumph of a two-pronged economic argument aimed at making US health care more efficient. On the one hand, requiring everyone to obtain health insurance makes risk pools larger and actuarially more predictable, reducing the need for surplus premiums as a cushion against unexpected risks. On the other hand, ensuring that everyone has secure access to routine and preventive care helps avoid the inflated costs of emergency care and delayed treatment.

These arguments advance the policy value of economic efficiency. For GBIO members the individual mandate is instead a matter of covenantal solidarity. The mandate assumed this participant value through GBIO's social actions, the most important of which was its affordability workshops. A Jewish organizer recounted how participants spilled their lives onto a form tallying up the items in their budget. On the front of the form, people listed their necessities—"heat, electric, food, child care, car insurance, and gas, not even other things like taking your kids to the movie." Participants talked back to the form, insisting that some of the optional expenses on the back side of the form—debt payments, monthly savings, tithing—should be listed as basic expenditures. The organizer continued that people "were deflated because it's depressing to look at their realities. Which is sort of perfect, right, because it's an action on all of us. Well, we know that our financial situations in our lives are challenging." The question is how to respond as a group to the competing pulls of family budgets and mandated coverage. Then the organizer named solidarity as the commitment that workshop participants took on themselves: "It's really about solidarity. Five hundred, six hundred of us are doing this, and then we're going to have a conversation with the Connector about what our lives say. . . . Most people felt like they were willing to pay something; they felt it was a responsibility."

When presented to the Connector Board, the data put faces to a debate about numbers, pressuring board members to set more forgiving affordability levels than the board's economist had proposed. When I asked about the significance of GBIO's presence at the meeting, observers disagreed. Was it a case of effective political pressure, as a consumer advocate characterized it, or was it a "moral force" that shifted the context of public deliberation, as a Jewish health policy expert on GBIO's leadership team described it?

Evidence for a changed moral context comes from Hamilton's posts on the second and third years of the affordability debate. As noted above, the second anniversary post opened with the epigraph "Mercy and truth are met together." Hamilton's exegesis starts with the participant value of truth: "Truth demands that we understand the necessity for an affordability schedule which holds individuals responsible for ensuring their own health—and we do."[34] This affirmation reflects a concession made, enacted, and embraced. Having accepted the individual mandate, first as a policy compromise and then through the work of its affordability workshops and enrollment canvassing, GBIO endorses it here. The mandate's rationale shifts, however, from individual responsibility for the sake of economic efficiency to individual responsibility for the sake of social solidarity. As this important distinction underscores, the policy language we apply to the individual mandate dictates the public questions we ask. If economic efficiency is the operative value, then the question is, What market structures and funding levels are required to make the system work efficiently? Where solidarity prevails, the question becomes, How should we calculate a person's or a family's fair share contribution to the social good of health care?

For Hamilton the biblical response is clear. If the value of truth means accepting individual responsibility for ensuring one's health, then mercy requires moderating annual increases in the affordability schedule. Increases can match the rise in the federal poverty level but not extract a growing percentage of people's income. In addition to staking this moral claim, Hamilton argues that the policy goal of keeping the system working efficiently implicates the economics of the individual mandate in precisely this kind of unfair income extraction. Taking the most obvious rejoinder first, Hamilton warns that if "the prices insurance companies want to charge" are allowed to set the schedule, then this "would signal that business profit and market greed are free to drive public policy."[35]

Hamilton returns to the economics of the individual mandate in year three when the Connector Board was weighing two new proposals for increasing premiums set by the schedule: (1) a 2 percent increase at all income levels or (2) a

2 percent increase below 300 percent of FPL and a 5 percent increase above that level. GBIO favored the shared responsibility of the first proposal, and they rejected the two different rationales offered for the counterproposal.

The first rationale in favor of the two-tiered increase was the concern with "crowding out" employer-sponsored insurance. If the state held premium increases to 2 percent while employer premiums soared at rates of 5 percent and higher, there would be perverse economic incentives for employers to dump their covered employees onto the Health Connector's insurance exchange. Simple economics, it seemed, required the 5 percent premium increases on higher-income earners or else companies would be compelled to heed their bottom line and drop employee coverage. Yet Hamilton notes that fears of crowding out employer-sponsored insurance had not materialized in previous years. In fact, more employers committed to offering their employees insurance, strongly suggesting that shared responsibility for the social norm of coverage for all Massachuestts residents was taking hold.[36] Hamilton anticipates that this social norm would trump the market incentive to drop insurance yet again. The second rationale for the two-tiered increase was the state's rising budget as it dealt with high health care inflation. Again simple economics requires increased revenues to offset budget overruns. "At first glance," Hamilton writes, "this seems to be a sound fiscal argument; however, it is important to remember that the Affordability Schedule is not just a *suggestion*. It is the standard that is used to *require* consumers to purchase health insurance; therefore [it] must, as near as possible, reflect the ability of consumers to pay the cost of their health insurance in the context of their real budgets not based on the price of the product or market trends."[37] The final line of this passage makes the key point. The price that private insurers and providers want to charge for their products hardly seems like a fair way to set a public policy as consequential as the affordability schedule. Nevertheless, market trends in insurance premiums and health care costs are the implicit measure in both of these economic rationales—against crowding out employer-sponsored insurance and against busting the state's budget.

Hamilton demonstrates how ostensibly neutral appeals to economic efficiency are linked to the unfair premise that prevailing market prices determine health care affordability. From the standpoint of efficiency, if premiums have to rise in state-sponsored programs to avoid giving employers incentives to drop employee coverage, then these premium hikes must be declared affordable. Similarly, if health care inflation empties the state's coffers, then affordability caps must rise commensurately. In short, as long as efficiency remains the operative priority, the affordability debate will keep circling back to a justice-in-exchange model that will be unfair and unsustainable as it squeezes people subject to the individual mandate past their breaking point. From the perspective of economic cost-benefit analysis, it makes sense to increase the burdens on mandated individuals given their benefit gains. Commutative justice prevails here. GBIO counters that solidarity requires other citizens to match the sacrifices of those citizens who have stepped forward under the individual mandate.

Something funny happened on the way to implementing the individual mandate. Once a reluctant policy compromise, the mandate was redefined through GBIO's community activism as a double expression of solidarity—first, by the affected residents' commitment to pay their portion and, second, in a more tentative return commitment by the state and its citizens to do their part in keeping mandated coverage affordable. Thus the participant values of truth and mercy reoriented the policy goal from efficiency to solidarity. Efficiency still matters to health care reform, but now it matters for the sake of health care solidarity. Cost savings are imperative so that expanded coverage remains affordable for all citizens.

THE POLITICS OF THE INDIVIDUAL MANDATE: LIBERTY OR DIGNITY?

Recasting the individual mandate as an expression of solidarity has a further consequence of blunting the objection that a publicly subsidized expansion of health coverage creates harmful new entitlements. Here we arrive at the political challenge confronting liberal arguments for positive rights to health care. Just as economic analysis has a hard time escaping arguments about efficiency that impose unfair standards of affordability, liberal policy arguments are easily tripped up by the cultural bias that assigns to the supposedly "undeserving poor" the moral laxity of feeling "entitled" to health care.

Underlying this objection to new entitlements is a political model of a just meritocracy. In this justice-in-exchange model, health coverage is earned through a job productive enough to merit insurance benefits as contracted by employer and employee. Senior citizens with a lifetime of work and politically contracted Medicare contributions can claim their rightful benefits too. There is also room for the disabled, and possibly children, to receive public support, as they are without fault in this merit-based social contract. As discussed in chapter 1, this contractual system of individual merit remains the dominant moral language of health care in United States. At the other end of the political spectrum, single-payer liberals would do away with the complex financing structure of private insurance, Medicare, and Medicaid, replacing the multiple avenues into US health care with a government health plan for everyone. In this liberal model of positive rights to health care, the respective standards of contributive and distributive justice are graduated tax payments and equal health benefits. For single-payer liberals the individual mandate falls woefully short of health care justice and may precipitate a backlash against truly universal coverage.

Despite the force of this argument, the political challenge facing advocates of a national health plan is profound and, in my judgment, culturally insurmountable in the "land of liberty." The politics of the individual mandate in Massachusetts is a case in point. One of the arguments for setting relatively high affordability standards was that a new entitlement to subsidized health coverage, without sufficient pain to people's income, would produce the "moral hazard" of overusing health care, bankrupting the commonwealth's treasury.

Instead of citing biblical values, Hamilton reframed the politics of the individual mandate using the gospel story of the widow's mite. He offered a narrative counterpoint to the American story of the socially productive and personally disciplining nature of market freedom: "Jesus sat down opposite the place where the offerings were put and watched the crowd putting their money into the temple treasury. Many rich people threw in large amounts. But a poor widow came and put in two very small copper coins, worth only a fraction of a penny. Calling his disciples to him, Jesus said, 'I tell you the truth, this poor widow has put more into the treasury than all the others' (Mark 12:41–43, NIV)."[38] The claim that the poor widow's coins amount to more than rich people's sums makes no sense in a commutative justice framework where one gets back commensurate with what one put in. It works only in a social justice framework where relative social standing matters morally. Recall that the participants in GBIO's affordability workshops insisted that tithing was a necessary, not an optional, expense. Their claim was a claim about dignity—that contributing one's gifts to a community is an essential part of human dignity. If tithing were foreclosed by the imposition of higher affordability standards, then people's sense of their own dignity would suffer.

Hamilton's story of the widow who gives her last coins upends the allegation that poor people are getting too much health care for too little, a clear violation of justice in exchange. Do people with private health benefits not feel "entitled" to their health care when the price exceeds their premiums? Who runs up the highest charges from overtreatment, patients in means-tested programs like Medicaid or the worried well with private insurance and Medicare? Such questions stand little chance of being aired in response to angry charges that new entitlements and taxes infringe on personal liberty. Arguments for positive rights to health care operate in the same orbit of personal liberty, so they struggle for liftoff. Although as a single-payer system answers to the policy values of shared responsibility and human dignity, it is justified in the language of individual rights. By contrast, GBIO's religious arguments shift the moral focus away from individual rights to health care for the sake of liberty to a shared responsibility for health care for the sake of dignity.

By clothing the individual mandate in the widow's dignity, Hamilton recasts the policy language and the public question yet again. He invokes the authority of Jesus and the practice of tithing to reorient a politics of resentment over other people's entitlements toward an ethics of respect for everyone's contributions to the social good of health care. Given the expense of even the subsidized coverage and the copays in the new Massachusetts plans, which is more worthy, Hamilton asks, the proverbial widow's mite under the individual mandate or the higher taxes paid by the affluent to keep the mandate affordable? Thus he draws a substantial portrait of the dignity of those who comply with the individual mandate and blunts the image of complacent vice that lurks at the bottom of American notions of meritocracy.

In just three years, the individual mandate led almost 200,000 Massachusetts residents to pay at least a portion of their new coverage. Beyond their financial contributions to the state's health care treasury, the newly insured have developed a leavening sense of deserved entry at the front door of the health care system, according to a Connector Board member I interviewed. As the value of dignity takes hold among the new policyholders, they are, in her words, teaching "hospitals to treat people with more respect because they can go somewhere else." Moreover, if the widow can sacrifice to pay for her mandated coverage, then businesses, insurers, hospitals, and physicians can sacrifice, too, by funding expanded coverage and by holding down the cost of quality care.

Here we return to the fundamental challenge to Chapter 58 and the ACA posed by market reformers: cost control. Previously I mentioned Tom Miller's criticism of Chapter 58 as crippled by the accumulation of regulations preceding it and by the public mandates and oversight built into it. Instead, Miller argues, Americans need two market tools essential to personal liberty: (1) transparent information about the health care expenditures made on their behalf and (2) personal choice among a wide array of deregulated health plans covering only those health care services that consumers want for their money. As we have seen, in theory market reform promotes the twin principles of consumer choice and personal responsibility to drive down health care costs. In reality, the force of these two principles cuts in different directions. If market reform were adopted as the savior of the health care system, then the benefits of consumer choice would mostly flow to the wealthy and the healthy, while charges of personal irresponsibility would largely redound to the poor and the sick (see chapter 5).

By applying the story of the widow's mite to the individual mandate, Hamilton disrupts the reinforcing loop of consumer choice and individual merit in the market reformers' vision of contributive and distributive justice. The loop begins with the idea that health coverage and health care are private goods that consumers ideally purchase for themselves, using their own resources or funds from an employer or the government. In addition, consumers who take the time to investigate insurance and treatment options and to invest in wellness merit the payback of reduced premiums and expenditures. In sum, affordable health coverage and quality care are rightly distributed to those who contribute, first, through productive employment or Medicare taxes, and second, through healthy personal choices and discerning consumption of health care services. Those who put in deserve to get back. Although market reformers predict that affordable coverage and care will spiral out to others in the future, the immediate thrust of their argument justifies some people's lack of coverage and greater exposure to cost as the just consequences of insufficient personal responsibility and consumer initiative. GBIO's participant values of shared responsibility and solidarity reveal the one-sided respect for dignity *and* liberty implicit in relying on a vanguard of elite consumers to control health care costs.

According to GBIO, moving toward cost-effective delivery of care requires all stakeholders to join in solidarity at the policymaking table and be ready to make some sacrifices. Moreover, if every Massachusetts resident committed to healthier personal habits and a more cost-effective delivery system, the community would be enriched, even as a trimmer health sector would shed jobs, reduce salaries, and eliminate profitable but less effective treatments and procedures. That is not to say that GBIO is naive about the challenges. As the Jewish health policy expert on their leadership team observed, in pushing for more access, "we've been aligned with the hospital, and all of a sudden if you're really talking the cost issue, we've got to go after them because they are very much part of the problem." The question is, "Can you organize masses of people especially when some of the people sitting in those churches and synagogues earn their livings off the largesse of the health care system?" If ever there was a time to keep decision makers at the table in a spirit of solidarity, the cost control issue is it, as I address in the book's conclusion.

THE ETHICS OF THE INDIVIDUAL MANDATE

My argument for GBIO's vision of the individual mandate is more cultural than philosophical. In the absence of a basic solidarity in health care, neither the economic argument for efficiency through government regulation nor the liberal argument for positive rights to health care can win the reform debate in the United States. Strong liberal and economic arguments have long been offered in support of universal health coverage, but they have been hampered by the lack of solidarity in American political culture. GBIO's conversion to and conversion of the individual mandate through its participant values signal how this policy compromise can become the moral linchpin of a socially just American health care system.

The name of the individual mandate classifies it as a curious hybrid specimen. It is part creature of individual choice and part creature of government coercion. Unlike a single-payer system, individuals are free to choose their health plan in the private insurance market. Unlike market reform, that purchase of insurance is enforced and supported by the government. We can view the individual mandate as nothing more than a public regulation of private choice, or we can see it as a social arrangement for advancing a fuller solidarity behind the social good of US health care. The second approach is admittedly a difficult fit with American political culture, as can be seen in the three judicial opinions from the US Supreme Court's ruling in favor of the ACA.

The opinions align with the now familiar visions of health care justice discussed in this book. First, Justice Antonin Scalia's dissenting opinion conforms to the voluntary transactions of justice in exchange. His market-oriented opinion separates the health insurance market from the health care market. Congress created a free-rider problem through public policies that guarantee emergency access to the uninsured. The uninsured can ride for free, and it does not matter if they do so out of economic hardship or out of the economic calculation that their health risks do not merit the cost of health coverage. These people are "inactive" in the health insurance market, so there is no "activity" for Congress to regulate under the Constitution's Commerce Clause.[39]

Second, Chief Justice John Roberts's majority opinion echoes this reasoning but adds a minimalist social contract that justifies requiring uninsured Americans to pay a tax as a quid pro quo for guaranteed emergency access. In enacting the mandate, Congress recognized that the public pays the high cost of uncompensated care. So using its constitutional powers, Congress may "tax" uninsured people who ride for free. Roberts's position hews to Scalia's economic description of individuals choosing to remain "inactive" in the health insurance market, while also granting a limited obligation to contribute to a health care system from which everyone can expect some benefit.[40]

Finally, Justice Ruth Bader Ginsburg's concurring and dissenting opinion points to the social structures that currently finance uncompensated care in the

United States. The federal emergency access law, public funding of safety-net hospitals, and cost-shifting by insurers and providers speak to the high cost that some people's lack of insurance has for other Americans. As a result, choosing not to buy health insurance is not economic inactivity with no bearing on interstate commerce. It imposes tax and premium burdens on other Americans, directly affecting interstate commerce and justifying the individual mandate under the Commerce Clause.[41]

Although Ginsburg voted with Roberts's majority ruling, her vision of justice lost in this case. Fundamentally, Roberts affirmed the court minority's restriction of health care justice to the voluntary transactions that Americans choose to make with insurers and providers. Beyond these voluntary contracts, health care justice extends only into a minimalist social contract of guaranteed emergency care backed by a tax penalty on any American who "chooses" to remain uninsured.

The ACA's constitutionality stands on Roberts's reasoning. More noteworthy, however, eight of the nine Justices rejected his minimalist version of a health care social contract. Four conservatives would ban the individual mandate as an unwarranted federal intrusion on market choice. For them even a minimalist federal social contract offends personal liberty. Four liberals would affirm the individual mandate as a legitimate regulatory fix that helps rebalance shared responsibilities in the markets for health insurance and health care. For them the individual mandate is one more building block in a policy framework of shared responsibility.

The ACA seeks to build on existing social structures: (1) Medicaid shifts from a social welfare program to a social guarantee for the poorest Americans; (2) the individual mandate requires tens of millions of Americans to contribute through new premiums or taxes; (3) the employer mandate obliges firms with fifty or more full-time employees to contribute premiums or penalties; (4) federal subsidies reduce premium, deductible, and copay costs for individuals and families earning up to 400 percent of FPL who purchase a policy through the state insurance exchanges; (5) community rating lowers premiums for the sickest and oldest Americans; (6) adult children under age twenty-six can remain on their parents' policies, easing the burden on the young; (7) guaranteed issue of health insurance policies protects sick Americans from coverage denials for preexisting conditions; (8) the elimination of annual and lifetime caps on insurance payouts helps stave off medical bankruptcy; and (9) the annual review of private insurers' rate increases and the required minimum medical-loss ratios curb insurance profits. In addition to the goal of making affordable coverage more widely available, other provisions aim to ensure that this coverage is creditable: (1) the minimum essential coverage provisions set a baseline of services for quality coverage, and (2) the health insurance exchange's required consumer protections and transparency standards set a bar for insurers inside and outside the exchanges.

Shared responsibility cannot stop at policy design, however. Liberals who place their faith either in regulating the economics of US health care or in legislating a right to health care should heed the cautionary tale of the Supreme Court's narrow ruling. More important than the narrowness of the vote is the narrowness of Roberts's reasoning. His minimalist social contract may have saved the ACA from premature death, but it is too narrow a basis for the ACA's legitimacy and success. The deeper lesson of this case is that policy efforts aimed at strengthening the social good of US health care confront powerful political and economic beliefs reinforced by American institutions and culture. Although the federal government pours money into health care, its regulatory power over commerce must be constitutionally checked. Although uninsured individuals have guaranteed emergency access, their personal liberty must be protected in the insurance market. Although public funding is essential to medical research and training, market choice is the only route to high-quality care. These articles of faith in the limits of federalism, the supremacy of liberty, and the efficiency of markets are so potent that moving toward a socially just American health care system will take equally evocative visions of a community responding to shared vulnerability, backed by organizations putting their beliefs into action.

A comment by the rabbi on GBIO's leadership team cuts to the heart of the issue. As he put it, GBIO's purpose is to "speak the language of covenant in a contract-driven society." In the United States, he continued, "the dominant culture is a market-driven consumer model. Our organization is an engine for citizenship and community, and we leverage congregations, the best example of a covenantal community that we have." Liberal arguments for greater efficiency and more expansive liberty through universal coverage tend to operate in a contractual mode, too. If all Americans have coverage, then a more rational system can lower costs for everyone. If every American enjoys the right to health care, then the freedom to participate in society will be greatly enhanced. These arguments are fine as far as they go, and I hope their predictions prove true. But there will be many bumps along the way, as evidenced by the economics and the politics of the individual mandate in Massachusetts. Navigating those obstacles at the national level will require ensuring that the quest for efficiency serves health care solidarity and that the protection of liberty does not erase people's dignity.

In my judgment, moving the minimalist social contract of US health care toward a fuller covenant and common good will take religious congregations and interfaith coalitions bringing their values to the public debate. The common commitment to healing as a shared responsibility means that every congregation should have something to contribute. Often, these values will be stated in the biblical language or traditional beliefs of an insider community, and GBIO's values share this insider quality. Not only are they articulated in biblical terms, but they are also made meaningful through the experiential knowledge of a moral community. These two marks against GBIO's values hardly fit the moral philosopher and political liberal John Rawls's test of reciprocity. For Rawls and many secular liberals, political arguments about "constitutional essentials" and "matters of basic justice" must be articulated in terms that any reasonable citizen could reasonably accept.[42] I argue, however, that it is the participant character of GBIO's values that makes them both reasonable and compelling.

Grounded in participant values, GBIO's religious arguments matter less at the level of conclusion than motivation. They are less an appeal for assent than a call to action. Just as the core values of religious health care nonprofits must be articulated in operational and delivery structures that we can evaluate publicly and practically, so too GBIO's participant values are publicly accessible and practically assessable. They are already internally shared values, the product of an activist group's moral commitments, experiential lessons, community activities, and public arguments. They can be shared by any outsider willing to enter into these formative moral commitments and experiential lessons, at least imaginatively. How will people facing the individual mandate afford coverage? What response might other Americans make to honor this act of dignity? GBIO's religious values of dignity, justice, mercy, truth, compassion, shared sacrifice, stewardship, civility, noncomplicity, and solidarity will assume full meaning, however, only for those Americans motivated to act upon them in taking the ACA from a policy structure of shared responsibility to a cultural recognition of covenantal solidarity in health care.

Health care reform is a signal moment when progressive religious values might resurface in American public life. GBIO's activities generated grassroots solidarity and its participant values and public liturgy articulated a sophisticated covenantal ethics. Even as the democratic tradition in the United States tends to separate public arguments from religious values, GBIO's story demonstrates that there is room for cross-fertilization. In fact, cross-fertilization by religious convictions and moral languages is one of the most potent ways that the terms of American democracy have been rewritten historically. GBIO's interfaith activities and participant values are a model for churches, synagogues, mosques, and other religious groups to continue the work of health care reform nationally.

NOTES

1. In Nov. 2012, 48.5 percent of Americans viewed the ACA unfavorably (versus 42.3 percent favorably) (www.realclearpolitics.com/epolls/other/obama_and_demo crats_health_care_plan-1130.html#polls [accessed Nov. 12, 2012]). Some of this opposition reflected liberals' support for a public-option health plan or a single-payer health plan. See Saks, "What Do Polls Really Tell Us."

2. Religious arguments for solidarity in US health care appear in US Conference of Catholic Bishops, "A Framework for Comprehensive Reform"; Zoloth, *Health Care and the Ethics of Encounter*; and Townes, *Breaking the Fine Rain of Death*.

3. For state coverage, see Massachusetts Division of Health Care Finance and Policy, "Health Insurance Coverage in Massachusetts," 8. For national coverage, see Kaiser Family Foundation, "Health Insurance Coverage of the Total Population."

4. Long et al., "Massachusetts Health Reforms," 3.

5. Ibid., 5.

6. Massachusetts Division of Health Care Finance and Policy, "Massachusetts Employer Survey 2010," 6.

7. Massachusetts Health Connector, "Health Reform Facts and Figures" (Fall 2012), 3; www.mahealthconnector.org/portal/site/connector/menuitem.d7b34e88a23 468a2dbef6f47d7468a0c (accessed Oct. 26, 2012).

8. Long et al. "Massachusetts Health Reforms," 4–5.

9. Massachusetts Health Connector, "Health Reform Facts and Figures" (Fall 2012), 4.

10. Long et al. "Massachusetts Health Reforms," 6.

11. Ayanian and Van der Wees, "Tackling Rising Health Care Costs in Massachusetts," 791.

12. Miller, "Massachusetts," w452. A different explanation of the high cost of health care in Massachusetts emphasizes the high concentration of teaching hospitals (Wallack et al., "Massachusetts Health Care Cost Trends Part 1").

13. Woolhandler and Himmelstein, "The New Massachusetts Health Reform," 19–21.

14. I have followed Rev. Hamilton in listing the Bible translation whenever he provides one for his scriptural epigraphs. Otherwise he uses the Revised Standard Version.

15. Hamilton, "This Is the Day the LORD Has Made."

16. Cahill, *Theological Bioethics*, 38.

17. Ibid., 24.

18. Hamilton, "Why Outreach and Enrollment Matters."

19. Ibid.

20. I thank the anonymous reviewer who brought this double etymology of liturgy to my attention and suggested it as a framework for analyzing GBIO's public arguments.

21. Hamilton, "Come Now, and Let Us Reason Together."

22. Hamilton, "Health Care Reform: Where Do We Go from Here?"

23. Hamilton, "A Dying Hope on Easter Sunday Morning."

24. Hamilton, "Successful Implementation Requires Real Outreach and Enrollment."

25. Hamilton, "Truly Fair and Reasonable." Enrollment statistics are from Massachusetts Health Connector, "Health Reform Facts and Figures," 2009, 3; www.mass.gov/eohhs/docs/dhcfp/r/pubs/10/mes_aib_2009.pdf (accessed February 15, 2010).

26. Hamilton, "Continue to Care."

27. Hamilton, "A Call to Action!"

28. Hamilton, "What Is the Character of Our Commonwealth?"

29. Hamilton, "Give to Caesar, What Is Caesar's!"

30. Hamilton, "Walking through the Valley of the Shadow of Death."

31. Hollenbach, *The Common Good and Christian Ethics*, 195–97.

32. Ibid., 195–203.

33. Cahill identifies economics, liberalism, and science as three ostensibly "neutral" vocabularies that dominate public debates about bioethics. In her words, "The challenge before theologians [entering the public debate] is not to cast aside a thin discourse for a richer one, but to dislodge the thick discourses that are so widely entrenched that their constituting narratives and practices are no longer directly observed" (*Theological Bioethics*, 27).

34. Hamilton, "Continue to Care."

35. Ibid.

36. Massachusetts Division of Health Care Finance and Policy, "Massachusetts Employer Survey 2010," 6.

37. Hamilton, "Responding to the Signs of the Times."

38. Quoted in Hamilton, "Truly Fair and Reasonable."

39. Justice Antonin Scalia, "Dissenting Opinion," *National Federation of Independent Businesses v. Sebelius*, 10–16.

40. Chief Justice John Roberts, "Majority Opinion," *NFIB v. Sebelius*, 35–38. That Roberts presupposes a commutative justice framework is particularly clear in pages 24–27.

41. Justice Ruth Bader Ginsburg, "Concurring and Dissenting Opinion," *NFIB v. Sebelius*, 3–12.

42. Rawls, "The Idea of Public Reason Revisited," 575–78; and "The Idea of Public Reason," 215–18.

Conclusion
RELIGIOUS VALUES AND COMMUNITY CARE

There's a growing consensus that we have enough money in the health care system. Improving health care is about utilization, it's about delivery, it's about allocation of resources. When you get down to it, decisions in those areas are oftentimes value based. So I think Catholic health systems are uniquely positioned to talk about values, and not only uniquely positioned, but morally obligated to step up their level of advocacy. If these values that we have on our business cards have meaning, then there is a unique responsibility of big systems with the resources to go out and share.

> Director of state government relations,
> nationwide Catholic hospital system

HEALTH CARE WORKS only if everyone is in it together. This simple slogan is the crux of the argument in this book. To the credit of the legislators who wrote the Affordable Care Act, the law attempts to remedy many of the ways that US health care has fallen short of a system in which everyone is in it together. At the same time, the law's complexity highlights the deceptive simplicity of this slogan. There will be significant challenges on the road to an inclusive, fair, efficient, and sustainable health care system.

Among the most important challenges is cost control. Two statistics indicate why cost control is likely to drive much of the reorganization of US health care in the coming decades. The Centers for Medicare and Medicaid Services project that health care spending will rise to one-fifth (19.8 percent) of gross domestic product in 2020.[1] The Congressional Budget Office predicts that mandatory federal spending on Medicare, Medicaid, and the ACA's insurance subsidies will absorb 9 percent of the national economy by 2035, severely constraining other government services.[2] Statistical projections signal the urgency of cost control, but they offer no guidance about how to control costs while serving other health care values.

Oregon has a history of Medicaid reform that helps predict the broader effects of the ACA's extension of health coverage to low- and middle-income Americans. In 2008, the state had surplus Medicaid funds and held a lottery for new recipients. This randomized experiment created an ideal laboratory for health economists studying the benefits and costs of expanding Medicaid. The early lessons confound both sides in the national debate. Conservatives criticize Medicaid for its supposedly poor health outcomes. After the first year, however, new Medicaid enrollees reported improved health and even larger gains in happiness due to their relief at having coverage and their sense of belonging to the health care system. Liberals predict that guaranteeing access for everyone will lower the system's costs by avoiding the expense of delayed and emergency care. At least in the short run, however, new enrollees in Oregon's Medicaid program are using more services and increasing system costs.[3] The same pent-up demand for health care services is likely in the case of the newly insured enrollees in state health insurance exchanges. Thus the ACA's commitment to social inclusion will probably both improve newly insured people's health and cost Americans more in the coming years.

Better health for more people at a higher cost for more people: It is difficult tradeoffs like this that make the reform debate so fraught with tension. Competing values are in play, and they seem to diverge irreconcilably. What, then, gives the director of state government relations, quoted in this chapter's epigraph, the confidence that these value tensions could be resolved if religious health care organizations brought their core values to the health care reform debate? He claims that better health care can be attained at current funding levels. The question is how such values-driven decision making might transpire.

Once again, Oregon's Medicaid experiments are instructive. In the late 1980s and early 1990s, the state attempted to expand the number of people covered by Medicaid even as the state budget declined. Initial attempts were driven by a utilitarian logic of improving health outcomes for the largest number of residents. Legislators used the blunt instrument of cutting Medicaid funding for complex organ transplants, where life expectancy and expected post-operation quality of life were relatively low. They redirected funding to prenatal care, where the benefits for pregnant women and their babies were predictably high and lifelong. I will return to the public backlash that met this first step.[4] The state's next steps offer a fuller picture of what values-driven deliberation looks like as a political process.

State officials turned to a decade-old grassroots initiative of citizen dialogues called the Oregon Health Decisions project. All across the state, Oregonians were invited to articulate what health meant to them and which values should guide the allocation of health care services. This remarkable exercise in participatory democracy yielded six shared values, as summarized by Jewish ethicist Laurie Zoloth: "responsibility and limits, quality of life, longevity and meaning, greatest good for the greatest number, equity, and public good." Working from these values and within existing budgets, state officials created a list of 567 treatments that would be fully covered for an expanded number of Medicaid recipients. Treatments were ranked based on their medical efficacy in relation to the six values embraced by the citizen participants. Below treatment 567, no other services would be covered (transplants were to be covered). Although the full list of covered services exceeded federal Medicaid mandates, it was incomplete. The public outcry—in this case, mostly from outside the state—was intense. The administration of Pres. George W. Bush denied the waivers necessary to allow the experiment to proceed.[5]

Oregon's political experiment was participatory and largely consensual. It was values driven and balanced. It yielded a generous list of benefits for an expanded number of Medicaid recipients. Yet it failed for at least two reasons. First, it was more an exercise in intellectual solidarity than social solidarity. The citizen participants and the state legislators were naming public values and drafting services lists that, for the most part, they did not have to live under themselves. Thus their commitment to extend meaningful health care to more low-income residents was morally strong but socially distant. Second, Americans remain deeply resistant to public mechanisms for setting health care priorities and implementing limits. Every scientific panel that recommends against current medical practice—for example, cutting back on screenings for breast cancer and prostate cancer—is met with vehement criticism.[6] Even the Medicare Independent Payment Advisory Board established by the ACA is resisted by Democrats who voted for the law.[7] The American political culture of personal liberty makes it unlikely that better health care value for the money will be achieved by means of the public allocation approach used in Oregon.

MARKET REFORM AND
INDIVIDUAL PREFERENCES

Political processes of debating, legislating, and implementing shared priorities and limits are not the only means Americans have for signaling what they value in health care. According to market reformers, Americans are prevented from using the most powerful mechanism at hand: a free market in which consumer choice, provider innovation, and insurer competition determine cumulative priorities and eliminate unwanted waste. The collective good is not the exclusive domain of legislative deliberation and public policy; markets allocate a society's resources by aggregating individual preferences under the constraints of scarcity. In other words, individual consumers can decide what they value within the limits of their budgets. In this approach, personal liberty is honored as consumers act on their particular values. Innovative providers respond directly to the myriad preferences of individual consumers. The private structure of US health care is freed from the supposedly "shared" public values enshrined in inefficient and unfair government regulation.

In contrast to a public allocation approach, market reformers advocate an individual preference approach to achieving better health care value for the money. Consider how this would apply to two of the main drivers of US health care costs: a growing population of elderly Americans and the arms race in technological investment.[8] Both factors converge in the rising costs of the federal Medicare program. One reason is that US law forbids Medicare from denying reimbursement because a treatment is not cost effective. Likewise, the ACA prohibits Medicare's new Independent Payment Advisory Board from making "any recommendation to ration health care . . . or otherwise restrict benefits."[9] We have already seen in chapter 3 how Medicare funding ramped up technological investment in hospital care in the name of equity for all senior citizens. But equity is not the only value served by rules that are partly the product of political compromises with physicians protecting their authority and with businesses seeking profitable new ventures. Market reformers would tackle both the high-minded profession of equity and the cost-inflating rule that turns Medicare into a bottomless purse. Why not allow individual seniors to take their guaranteed premium support and negotiate the health coverage and services that they value? If seniors value the latest, technology-intensive therapies, then the rising cost of care for this part of the population will be justified and increasingly paid for by the users. If not, then cost control will set in without the fear that government bureaucrats are rationing Medicare. Theoretically, individual consumers will "self-ration," paying for the care that they value—always, of course, within the limits of their financial means and their current budget priorities.

Here we return to the pivotal question of health care reform. Should health care be more an individual responsibility or a social responsibility? If individuals can be responsible for their own health care spending, then the free play of consumer preferences in the marketplace is a reasonable approach to arriving at the collective good of health care. Recall, however, all of the component parts of this good—excellent medical training, innovative medical research, a vast infrastructure of acute care hospitals housing much of this training and research, public insurance programs and private insurance pools supporting this infrastructure, public funding of uncompensated care, community benefits policies, community health centers taking primary care into underserved areas, and public health initiatives addressing the social harms of contagion and the social determinants of poor health. If health care is seen as a matter of individual responsibility, then instead of asking who is responsible for all of this health care spending, Americans can simply ask, What health coverage and health care services do I value for my money? In other words, the "our commitment" to fund the social good of US health care can be allowed to give way to the "my mentality" of market reform. Almost certainly, however, the shared values built into US health care would be lost from view and the supporting social structures would lose out on funding.

The likely consequences were summed up by a Baptist director of ethics and pastoral care at a nonprofit health care system in the Midwest. "Our economy has passed through the dot-com bubble and the housing bubble. Next up is the health care bubble." From his perspective, too much of health care is inflated. Acute care and specialty care remain patients' first resort and recoup the highest payments. Capital improvements in the fanciest facilities and redundant technology are going through the roof. Medical devices and pharmaceuticals command unjustifiably high prices. Health care job growth is too fast, and salaries outpace the broader economy. "Regardless of the reform path we choose," he predicted, "we are headed into an era of shrinking reimbursement. The air has to be let out of the balloon, but how will it come out? The Affordable Care Act buys time to let the air out more slowly." By contrast, market reform would pop the balloon, as "rational" consumers opt for overly lean health policies and cut back even on care for chronic conditions. With the balloon popped, health care options for the wealthy would initially shoot skyward while poorer Americans would see theirs fall. As individual payment took hold in what has become a heavily socially subsidized system, US health care would ultimately deflate to everyone's detriment.

This image accurately conveys the losses in equity and excellence that, in my judgment, would result from choosing the path of market reform. Expansion and equity have raced ahead of cost control in the public priorities of US health care, and market reformers target the public values written into US health policy as the cause. In response, they seek a health care system that answers directly to the values of individual consumers, but their envisioned system of private choice and private enterprise is at odds with the public-private partnerships that built and that sustain the social good of US health care. As should be clear by this point, not every aspect of this social good is good for our society. But instead of simply eliminating social investments in US health care, as market reformers propose to do, the better reform path joins social investment with social coordination. In writing the ACA, legislators avoided exclusive reliance on either the market coordination of individual preferences or the government coordination of public allocation. In place of these economic and policy mechanisms, American citizens are invited to step into the void and assume the shared responsibilities of social stewardship.

THE ACA AND SOCIAL STEWARDSHIP

Before explaining what I mean by social stewardship, let me acknowledge that the ACA answers to two other priorities first. The ACA's primary goals are lowering inequitable coverage barriers and increasing shared payments into US health care. Historically, three groups have faced unfair coverage barriers in the United States—the working poor, the sick and disabled, and the purchasers of individual coverage. First, health coverage has priced out tens of millions of working Americans who cannot afford their employers' coverage or buy a policy on their own. Indeed, work often does not pay in earning health benefits. In response to this reality, the ACA transforms Medicaid from traditional welfare "aid" to people who are incapable of working into a foundational guarantee for the working poor. Second, prior to the ACA, losing the social lottery of illness and disability could be made doubly painful by losing out on health coverage, too. In response to this double jeopardy, the ACA eliminates coverage denials for preexisting medical conditions and guarantees reissue of health policies to the sick and disabled. Finally, people who purchase insurance policies on their own have faced inflated premiums and out-of-pocket costs while also missing out on covered workers' tax advantages. In response to these burdens on the self-employed, the ACA's state health insurance exchanges enlarge risk pools to reduce average costs and add subsidies mirroring the tax deductions that covered workers have long enjoyed. This recompense is overdue.

In addition to greater equity in health coverage, the ACA extends shared payments into US health care through its individual and employer mandates. Much of the law's controversy revolves around these two mandates and the minimal essential coverage rules for most health policies. Uninsured Americans who are subject to the individual mandate now must pay into private insurance pools or into the federal health care budget. Employers with over fifty full-time employees face new "shared responsibility" penalties if they do not offer coverage or if their workers opt into a state health insurance exchange.[10] In this way the ACA acknowledges that greater equity in coverage requires greater equity in sharing health care costs. Individuals and employers who have ridden the system for free, knowing that emergency care was always a fallback option, must now pay some of their freight.

Resistance to the mandates reflects more than economic hardship. As employers cut back on staff and staff hours in response to passage of the ACA, their announcements have been characterized more by indignation at government interference than by resignation at financial realities. The chorus of moral outrage will likely swell as individuals facing tax penalties on their 2014 federal forms decry this infringement of personal liberty. Clearly, more is at stake than economic regulations and policy structures. The ACA portends a change in consciousness. It upsets Americans' cultural expectations about health care. Specifically, the individual rights framework that liberals and conservatives have both brought to the reform debate gives way to the idea of health care as a social good. How exactly, Americans are likely to ask, does the individual mandate codify a right? Uninsured Americans now have the "right" to purchase health insurance or to pay a tax penalty? In reality, instead of codifying a right, the individual and employer mandates buttress an emerging social norm of expected coverage for all Americans. The law's other moving parts aim to ensure that this social norm is neither excessive in its individual burdens nor meaningless in its mandated benefits.

Cultural commitments to market freedom and personal liberty carry considerable moral force at present; thus the expectation that noncovering employers and uninsured Americans will contribute to the social good of health care is currently seen as an affront. Extrapolating from the experience in Massachuestts, however, I expect the onus of moral opprobrium to shift. The more that uncovered Americans step forward to purchase insurance under the individual mandate, the less patience there will be with those who complain about the relatively low cost of the ACA's tax penalties or with businesses that cut staff to avoid their fair share payments. The policy framework of the ACA adds to the existing social norm of guaranteed emergency care the complementary social norm of fair and reasonable contribution. Although important, this cultural change does not suffice by itself. If the ACA only increases funding into US health care by spreading the costs more equitably, then it will repeat the old policy story of the values of expansion and equity outpacing cost control once again (see chapter 3).

Yet cost control mechanisms are written into the ACA, and they represent a different approach than either the public allocations approach used in Oregon or the individual preferences approach of market reformers. The ACA approaches cost control in terms of social stewardship. "Social stewardship" involves managing costs by supporting those shared health care structures that extend wellness throughout communities and that enable wise personal decisions for the good of health. As an example, consider the ACA's requirement that health plans provide free preventive services. The economic incentive of free care should help Americans make the wise decision of establishing a relationship with a primary care doctor. The ACA also encourages social stewardship by changing the public financing of Medicaid, Medicare, community health centers, and community hospitals. As Medicaid becomes a safety-net guarantee, the ACA increases reimbursements for primary care to attract more physicians to low-income communities and to prioritize prevention and wellness. The ACA also ends the inflated subsidies that have been paid to privately run Medicare Advantage plans. In an era of cost control, private insurers must be as efficient as the government. The ACA's capital investments in community health centers support the shift from expensive emergency access to lower-cost routine care in the community. The law's reductions in disproportionate share hospital payments reflect this new priority of community wellness. At the same time, community hospital revenues are protected because the ACA disqualifies all new independent physician-owned hospitals from Medicare eligibility.

As this book has shown, the subtleties of federal financing remain out of public view, so these structural changes have largely gone unnoticed. Attention has focused more on Medicare's new Independent Payment Advisory Board (IPAB), which is, in fact, both advisory and independent. In its advisory capacity, the board's fifteen experts will study best practices for delivering quality care at lower costs and will encourage their adoption across the health industry. In its independent capacity, the board is charged with recommending a mandatory savings plan to Congress any year that Medicare exceeds spending targets. What makes the board independent is that Congress must accept its complete recommendations on a fast track or pass an alternative plan with equivalent savings.[11] Supporters view the board as a way to end lobbying pressure from special interests, while critics foresee a loss of public accountability and imminent rationing, despite the ACA's prohibiting IPAB from rationing care, altering Medicare benefits, or increasing beneficiaries' financial obligations. To operate within these limits, IPAB will have to focus on social stewardship—prioritizing lower-cost primary care and proactive chronic disease management and supporting personal decisions that minimize the risks of catastrophic care. Of course, as senior citizens near death, the only way to "avoid" the costs of catastrophic care is to decide against intensive lifesaving procedures, choices over which IPAB members have—and should have—no discretion.

Another ACA initiative invites social stewardship on a much broader basis. The private Patient Centered Outcomes Research Institute will sponsor, compile, and publicize comparative effectiveness research on the benefits and risks of medical procedures, tests, drugs, and devices. The institute has no power to determine coverage guidelines. Instead, it will be a clearinghouse of information for physicians and patients to use as they weigh the prices, risks, and outcomes of different treatment options. In a health care system where expansion and equity are the drivers, the newest technologies and the latest therapies become essential weapons in the arms race among providers for market share. At present the marketing of promised benefits goes unchecked in the vacuum left by a lack of trustworthy information about comparative effectiveness. The Patient Centered Outcomes Research Institute responds to these one-sided market forces, giving patients and their physicians a critical tool for pushing back and making medical decisions as citizens increasingly aware of shared health care costs. Certainly, patients must know the price of health care to engage in social stewardship. The high deductibles of market reform could contribute here in driving the hidden costs of health care out into the open for consumers to weigh as citizens.

Social stewardship makes cost control a shared responsibility among patients, providers, insurers, businesses, and governments. According to health policy experts John Mechanic, Stuart Altman, and John McDonough, this shared responsibility has taken hold in Massachusetts. In their words, "Massachusetts' experience demonstrates that the interplay between an active public policy and an engaged private sector can catalyze change more quickly than private or public action alone."[12] In this, the Massachusetts case helps anticipate future prospects for social stewardship.

Public-private partnerships are familiar in US health care, though putting them to work on cost control is not. Consider, first, the active public policy steps taken in Massachusetts. Just two years into the reform experiment, a 2008 law empowered the state to collect and review the charges on care billed by all of the leading providers in the state. Two years later, another law authorized the state to use this data to compare the relative value of providers' care. In addition to improving data collection on providers, the state has started denying individual- and small-group insurance premium rate hikes that they deemed unreasonable. Health insurers have also been required to offer at least one tiered health plan with cost reductions of 12 percent or more by taking advantage of a preferred list of in-network providers. Finally, State employees and participants in the Health Connector insurance exchange have received incentives to switch to these plans.

Turning to the private sector, Blue Cross Blue Shield of Massachusetts, the state's largest insurer, has initiated its new Alternative Quality Contracts with providers. Instead of paying for each service performed, these global payments for patient care give providers incentives to avoid medical errors, hospital readmissions, and costly long-term complications for their patients. The hard-charging private equity company Cerberus Capital has invested in information technology and community hospitals for its Steward Health System. Its goal is a provider network offering health care at a 15–30 percent discount outside of downtown Boston. Responding to these fiscal pressures from the state, from insurers, and from fellow competitors, provider organizations are taking cost-cutting steps throughout their operations.[13]

Massachusetts remains one of the highest-cost states for health care in the United States. The reasons include the state's leadership as a health care training and research hub as well as its high-income profile. With its 2012 cost control law, Massachusetts took three more steps aimed at bending the cost curve downward. First, the law sets an annual benchmark for health care spending across the state. From 2013 to 2018, spending increases cannot exceed the growth of the gross state product (GSP). For the next five years, the target falls to GSP minus 0.5 percent. In 2013, the allowed increase was 3.6 percent compared to an expected rise of 6.3 at the national level, demonstrating the cap's dramatic potential. Second, the law makes the state a leader in payment reform, requiring by 2015 that 80 percent of its Medicaid enrollees join health plans with global payments. Global payments cover the health of a population instead of the specific health care goods and services ordered for a patient. The incentive here is to keep people healthy within a global budget. Finally, the law creates a Health Policy Commission. Although the commission has limited enforcement powers, it represents the social coordination piece that has long been the missing complement to the social investment side of health care as a social good. As described by a Jewish health policy expert with the GBIO, the commission has the power to *frame* the public debate over cost control and *name* what the price and quality data say. The commission also has the power to *tame* and *shame* providers that exceed their billing allowance under the state's annual caps, and they can assign *blame* to any party driving excessive medical inflation, including patients themselves.[14] Viewing these public-private efforts as a whole, we see the economic values of efficiency, responsiveness, and transparency swinging into action in Massachusetts through social stewardship, not through the individual preferences of powerful consumers.

One tool of market reform, high-deductible health plans, will continue to spread, notably through state health insurance exchanges. If these plans are not used to punish poor people, who are perceived to be the problem, then consumer-directed care can help teach Americans to weigh the personal cost of unhealthy habits and to question their caregivers about the relative expense, benefits, and risks of different treatment options. But market reform will not get us to an efficient, responsive, and transparent health care system by itself. Market reform takes too narrow a view of these economic values. Efficiency in cost control is measured in local markets at facilities with very different public obligations and infrastructure costs. Responsiveness to consumer value is biased toward more affluent and better-insured patients. Transparency in price and quality is driven by competition for market share rather than by commitment to community health. The ACA expands these economic values into broader social measures. It supplements market-based efficiency measures with national research into best practices and comparative effectiveness. Its payment experiments with Accountable Care Organizations should help integrate care for Medicare patients. Its support of community health centers aims to do the same for low-income patients. Admittedly, the ACA offers little help with price transparency. Social stewardship relies on more than public policy, however. Insurance companies can prove their value to the health care system here. They have vast stores of pricing data, and they should help their members become smarter consumers. In addition, religious health care providers should assume moral leadership in publicizing clear price lists for all of their services.

The cost control measures written into the ACA and advanced in Massachusetts fit neither the public allocation approach used in Oregon's Medicaid program nor the individual preference approach championed by market reformers. Admittedly, these measures may prove insufficiently aggressive, lacking the teeth of either public enforcement or consumer discipline. Their success depends on something else—a new spirit of social stewardship in public-private partnerships coupled with broader social action and cultural change.

There are two important lessons here. First, many Americans still speak the language of health care as a private benefit, so naturally they see their salvation in private choice. Their assumptions conflict, however, with the country's long-standing reliance on social structures for sharing health care risks, costs, and benefits and with the history of social investments that have progressively made US health care into a social good. Second, these social investments have not been matched by social coordination. The ACA begins to integrate social coordination by mandating broader participation in funding the health care system and by establishing new tools for social stewardship. The ACA is congruent with the public-private partnerships that built US health care and the public values enshrined therein. It will take Americans investing themselves in these values and embracing the social good of US health care to flesh out the legislative skeleton of the ACA and start moving toward affordable, quality health care for all.

RELIGIOUS VALUES AND COMMUNITY ENGAGEMENT

The ACA invites a change in consciousness and a call to action. Even when grounded in thoughtful democratic reflection on values, policy structures are not enough for lasting health care reform. Earlier I mentioned the public backlash against Oregon's decision to stop covering complex transplants for Medicaid patients in order to extend its funding of prenatal care. Zoloth vividly describes the backlash as the media profiled Medicaid patients in need of a transplant and the public understandably identified with them, particularly with younger patients. People responded with charity collections at bake sales and grocery store checkouts.[15] This moral identification with people in health crisis mirrors the biblical models of healing discussed in chapter 2. The Torah teaches the duty of not standing idly by our neighbor's blood. The Good Samaritan reaches out and nurtures the neighbor back to health as wholeness. Where such direct actions are impossible, personal philanthropy expresses moral concern.

This personal moral identification and the philanthropy it engenders are praiseworthy. They have their limits, however, limits that obscure the social priorities of wellness, prevention, and cost-effective care for all Americans. The hard-won intellectual solidarity around Oregon's Medicaid expansion foundered on this personal moral identification with health crisis. A social solidarity is also needed to extend Americans' moral imagination beyond the acute care setting of medical heroism at death's door. An emergency ethics of survival at all costs must expand into a community ethics of wellness paid for together. I submit that religious providers and religious congregations have a vital role to play in getting people to explore the variety of values in US health care and working out their tensions in a balanced, fulsome way.

Two obstacles may short-circuit these conversations. Historically, when religious values have entered the debate, they have foregrounded the duties of lifesaving care at the expense of the broader social obligations of covenant and common good. The urgency and individualism of rights to health care only reinforce our national tendency to invest in the acute and specialized medicine delivered in the latest high-tech facilities—well after the fact of prevention, wellness, or chronic disease management. Politically, religious values are used to gain emotional support for one side of the debate or the other. Conservative appeals to the right to life sometimes cast liberals as callous toward human life. Superficial appeals to religious values can be found on the political left, too. Consider an example from my interviews: "Forget about the moral stuff; it's all about power." I heard this remark from the health policy expert from GBIO. He was relating the opinion of one of their coalition partners in the Massachusetts reform campaign, a former legislator who drew a sharp line between moral values in public discussions and political power in the policymaking process. For him the moral stuff only matters if it gains signatures on petitions, motivates demonstrators to march on the Capitol, or attracts the attention of journalists. Appealing to moral values is a matter of striking the right emotional chords in the public arena so that sufficient pressure is felt behind the closed doors of politics.

Liberals' dismissive attitude toward religious values in public policy is one of the reasons why Americans tend not to see health care reform as an ethical issue. Yet making the full range of values count in health care ethics is an urgent task moving forward. Why? Because the moral stuff *is* political power. I do not mean the way that politicians intone values in their sound bites. The important task is hammering out what health care values mean to different people and how they apply to concrete policies. Public deliberation and political legitimacy depend on working out the moral stuff. When the employees of religious health care organizations discuss their operations in light of their mission and values or when activists put their religious convictions into practice, two things can happen that give otherwise abstract values focused power and broad allegiance. First, when people decide organizational policies and plot strategic actions after reflection on their values, the consensus that arises through compromise is better defined and more sustainable. Second, these dialogue sessions and the actions that issue from them can energize and transform participants when they see their values refracted through other people's convictions and experiences. These twin dynamics of consensus through compromise and renewal through encounter give health care values their "moral stuffing." Together they also generate social solidarity.

Social solidarity requires identifying with people left out of health care, taking a stand alongside them as people deserving needed care, and joining in efforts to make theirs a situation one is willing to live with oneself. The easy solution of achieving greater equity at a higher cost no longer suffices. The priorities of social stewardship and healthy communities must take hold even as commitments to life-saving care and excellent medicine continue. Americans need to learn to live amid the tensions among health care values. As stated in the chapter's epigraph, religious providers should "go out and share" the full range of their core values. Ultimately, though, only religious congregations have the community presence and moral authority to inject social solidarity and social stewardship into health care reform on a national basis.

RELIGIOUS VALUES AND COMMUNITY CARE

Without a cultural transformation in how Americans perceive health care and their place in it, the ACA will not achieve the political legitimacy required to implement its provisions nor the community partnerships needed to slow rising health care spending. To borrow from medical ethicist Larry Churchill, it is time to move "beyond a sociality that is factual to one that is intentional."[16] Although Americans may not readily warm up to the idea that US health care already is a social good, the religious providers and interfaith activists profiled in the second half of this book offer rich vocabularies, backed by vivid imagery and visionary stories that speak to why our mutual vulnerability demands a communal response of covenant, common good, tzedakah, charity, and ministry. The words are as varied in their moral implications as the religious traditions from which they come, but the common thread among them is that healing is a shared responsibility.

Jim Strietelmeier, the minister at Neighborhood Fellowship in Indianapolis, whom I met after completing my interviews, described this common obligation provocatively. In his words, "Health care is a mercy not a right." Putting the mercy of health care before the right to health care shifts the action away from the government as the guarantor of rights and the individual claimants on this right. It relocates responsibility out beyond the hospital and the clinic and into a community's shared responsibilities. Mercy summons Americans to reflect and speak together in search of public agreements about how to respond to one another's health care needs within the limits of fiscal sustainability and human finitude.[17]

In the absence of social cooperation and civic trust around health care reform, there is little room to build the policy structures, take the organizational risks, establish the community partnerships, or the make shared sacrifices for comprehensive reform. Opponents can point to one threatened value among the many health care values and denounce the whole package. Even supporters can be one-sided in their good intentions. I close with three value tensions—mercy and truth, charity and justice, dignity and stewardship—that surround some of the most difficult issues that Americans will confront in the years ahead. I only trace these tensions and issues. Doing more would foreclose the congregational dialogue that breathes life into religious values. The power of consensus through compromise and the spark of renewal through encounter that arise from congregations navigating these value tensions are essential to naming and inspiring the makings of healthy communities.

MERCY AND TRUTH

The importance of mercy as a health care value reminds us of GBIO's efforts to balance mercy and truth in implementing the individual mandate in Massachusetts (see chapter 6). Against conservative critics of health care entitlements, GBIO president Rev. Hurmon Hamilton proclaimed the truth that individuals need to be held "responsible for ensuring their own health." The financial responsibilities assumed by low- and middle-income people under the individual mandate are a powerful rebuttal to conservative criticisms of "entitled" freeloading. Against budget-conscious liberal supporters of reform, Hamilton insisted on the mercy of keeping this mandated coverage affordable through shared sacrifice. If the only people sacrificing financially are those individuals subject to the mandate, then the social norm of expected coverage will be built on the backs of hard-pressed Americans.[18]

The reasonableness of the individual and employer mandates depends on Americans' taking ownership of and actively balancing the values of truth and mercy. The truth is that those individuals and businesses that have counted on the safety net of guaranteed emergency care should acknowledge that other Americans have been shouldering the burden of their health risks. At the same time, if Americans who already enjoy excellent health coverage, subsidized through tax advantages and Medicare benefits, are unwilling to make any sacrifices as the ACA is implemented, then they should be judged as lacking in mercy. From the Hebrew Bible comes the injunction, "You shall do no injustice in judgment; you shall not be partial to the poor or defer to the great, but in righteousness shall you judge your neighbor" (Lev. 19:15).

Religious congregations should support moral dialogue aimed at balancing truth with mercy. Impartiality means asking those members who are embittered by their new obligations under the ACA why they should not contribute to a social good that Americans pay for together. Instead of admonishment, moral support can be offered in the usual forms of prayer and liturgy timed to the civil New Year when the individual mandate began in 2014. Celebrating the shared benefits of US health care, acknowledging people's new financial responsibilities under the ACA, and committing to hearing and responding to anyone's financial struggles can generate a new openness inside congregations. A growing consensus around the truth that we pay for US health care together could yield greater willingness to contribute financially and to show mercy to fellow taxpayers by improving one's own health. Indeed, mercy is a two-way street. It is not simply a community supporting care for the needy regardless of the circumstances or their past behavior. It requires everyone taking care to keep health care costs down in the interests of a common good.

Truths about the personal responsibilities of paying one's part for health coverage and adopting healthy habits for everyone's benefit are difficult to speak out loud. Creating a space in which truths can be spoken and heard with mercy is more likely to begin inside congregations where moral exhortation and compassionate acceptance frequently mix. Learning about other people's struggles to meet their obligations under the mandates could help build public support for adequate subsidy levels and, possibly, new taxes to pay for them. Hearing how people are embracing healthier habits in their lives can inspire fellow congregants to join both in spirit and in activity. Activities might include community gardens, wellness walks, team weight-loss challenges, recreational sports, chronic disease support groups, or pitch-ins that feature a healthy recipe exchange and local experts providing information about accessing community health resources. Keeping activities fun helps acknowledge that mental, emotional, spiritual, and communal health are as vital as physical health. Humor helps, too: "God, bless this healthy food we eat today, teaching us to enjoy it as much as the fast food our processed taste buds love so well—and so ill." Speaking truth and responding with mercy are essential values for congregations to practice as communities committed to the abundance of health.

CHARITY AND JUSTICE

Since the founding of religious hospitals in the United States, charity care has been central to their mission. Through leadership and financial support, sponsoring religious orders and congregations made charity for poorer patients a principal expression of the mercies of health care. As religious providers have grown in size and autonomy, however, congregational focus on health care charity has shifted overseas. Even the amount of uncompensated care provided by religious hospitals should decrease with the ACA's coverage expansion. How then might congregations practice charity in US health care today? Alternatively, perhaps charity should give way to justice? In fact, there remains ample room for charity in US health care. By partnering with nonprofit providers and through interfaith coalitions, congregations can engage in charity with greater justice for all.

We can clarify the tensions between charity and justice by asking the question, Should there be any charity care in a just health care system? For some of my interviewees, the answer is an emphatic no. In the words of the government relations director at the Jewish hospital, charity care is such "a nineteenth-century concept. . . . The answer to the uninsured is to insure people." Similarly, a liberal Protestant member of GBIO argued that charity keeps us "distanced from the problem," whereas "justice is about saying that your problem is my problem. My problem is your problem. And we're going to fight together to solve that problem." In a conservative Protestant vision of a decent society, however, charity care for one's poor neighbor is an essential mercy that complements the justice of providing for one's family's health care. The Catholic vision of the common good includes charity care for the poor and vulnerable as intrinsic to health ministry. Although the root word *tzedek*, or justice, conveys the justice orientation of Jewish ethics, *tzedakah* includes financial assistance for poor people's health care.

The question of whether charity care belongs in a just health care system highlights important ethical differences among religious groups, but it remains a purely academic question in the United States. Under the ACA, four groups of people will still seek charity care. There will be millions of middle-income Americans who cannot afford their obligations under the individual mandate and millions more low-income Americans who reside in states that opt out of the Medicaid expansion. Undocumented immigrants will be uncovered because the ACA excludes them from participating in Medicaid and the state health insurance exchanges. Moreover, the ACA excludes all legal immigrants from Medicaid for five years but allows them premium credits in the insurance exchanges. This legal framework raises questions of justice: What is a fair and workable structure of subsidy support? What justifies states opting out of a Medicaid expansion that would serve millions of working Americans while being largely paid through the federal government? Is anything more than charity care owed to new legal immigrants or to the undocumented immigrants living and laboring among us?

Clearly the ACA anticipates the continuation of uncompensated care. These obligations will partly be met through the community benefits of nonprofit hospitals and the occasional care of free clinics. The provision of uncompensated care should shift, however, toward community health centers in tandem with the ACA's funding priorities of primary and preventive care. In striking the best balance, an urgent question is how charity care can be provided effectively without unjust burdens on taxpayers. Congregations can play a vital role here, as illustrated by an anecdote I heard while visiting a community health center. In front of the building was a bus stop with a line of people. My host related that patients often waited there for rides to the downtown public hospital where they sought care in the emergency department. The health center's efforts to bring these patients through their doors were frustrated by the force of habit, the cost of sliding-scale fees, and the wait for scheduled appointments. In helping to connect patients to community care, parish nurses and other health ministry volunteers should seek out members of their congregations who are shut out of health coverage, then explain their options for community care, and guide their transition into a relationship with a primary caregiver at a local health center. Expanding this charitable outreach, congregations could provide funding or apply for grants to defray health center fees. For their newly insured members, a church, synagogue, mosque, or temple could introduce mentoring programs, in which a practiced hand accompanied a novice on his or her journey into health insurance and the unfamiliar routines of preventive or chronic care. If extended beyond congregations and across class, racial, or ethnic lines, the moral and spiritual lessons from these encounters would likely flow back with greater force to the accompanying mentors, supplying added reasons for affluent congregations to embrace mercy at the next New Year's affordable health care liturgy.

In addition to congregant-to-congregant partnerships, congregations can form educational and collaborative partnerships with local providers. Mission-driven providers use orientation sessions to introduce new staff to their core values and sponsoring religious tradition. These sessions could be altered to instruct faith leaders about health care in their communities, stressing the sponsoring organization's successes *and* frustrations in meeting core values. The persistent need for charity care and unjust obstacles to good health would have to be central topics. Congregations in poorer areas have much to teach provider organizations here. The ACA requires nonprofit hospitals to conduct periodic community health needs assessments, and these congregations can speak directly to the challenges encountered by underserved groups of immigrants, non-English speakers, and other Americans whose health needs remain largely unheard.

Moving to collaboration would shift these conversations from identifying health needs toward mobilizing health assets. What community resources go unused? What working models might be adapted to different cultural and geo-graphic settings? How might hospital competitors coordinate services for under-served groups? Which impediments to better health do community members stress—transportation to and translation services at provider organizations, or malnutrition, pests, poverty, and violence in their neighborhoods? How might congregations, service providers, and health care providers partner to combine their assets for sustainable solutions? Simply put, how can "your" problem and capacities become "my" problem and "our" capacities? More direct partnerships could include provider organizations sponsoring health ministries within con-gregations. Health ministries lend nurturing relationships, community knowl-edge, and trusted advocacy to the clinical encounter between physician and patient.[19] Without trusting relationships nurturing healthy habits, even the best medical advice is unlikely to sustain the behavioral change required in chronic disease management. Neighborly care for recently hospitalized patients is often the best medicine for ensuring the kind of compliance that avoids a rapid return to the hospital and the cost it incurs. If congregations were essential partners in an accountable care organization structure, then nonprofit providers could fund their health ministries out of the payments received for avoided hospital read-missions and preventable catastrophic care.

The full promise of such congregation-provider partnerships is that charitable outreach becomes community exchange, with the potential to transform US health care toward greater justice—a fuller sharing in the benefits of better health and a decrease in the collective costs of paying for it. Interfaith collabora-tion across congregations can further this interweaving of charity with justice. Interfaith coalitions help simply due to scale. Provider organizations can partner more easily with a large coalition with more members and more extensive com-munity connections. More importantly, interfaith collaboration can mediate the theological pulls among congregations that understand and rank charity and justice differently. If conservative Christians engaged in these partnerships, then they would likely be more open to the importance of health care justice across different covenantal spheres, including the government's role in filling the gaps between family justice and congregational charity. If religious liberals joined, they would likely be moved into greater personal charitable outreach, acknowl-edging that investing in healthy communities takes more than advocacy for health care rights and health policy alone.

DIGNITY AND STEWARDSHIP

The final value tension is likely to be the most stubbornly contentious. The discomfort of truth and the sacrifice of mercy are personally difficult. Charity and justice divide communities theologically and politically. Through the sustenance of congregational life and the engagement of community partnerships, however, we can imagine balancing truth and mercy, charity and justice. By contrast, the suggestion that protecting human dignity be balanced with stewarding shared health care resources is anathema to some religious visions of life's meaning and the fundamental duties of healing. Dignity and stewardship collide most visibly in decisions about end-of-life care. A consistent indicator of this conflict is that one-quarter of Medicare spending on the elderly covers patients in the final year of their life.[20]

From the national debate over the ACA to public battles over continuing life support in cases like Terri Schiavo's, Americans are familiar with religious objections to rationing or otherwise ending life-saving care for terminally ill or dying patients. Nevertheless, I propose that politics and culture are greater impediments than religion to balancing dignity with stewardship. Putting health care mercies before health care rights is especially important here.

In my judgment, using rights to navigate the coming value conflicts between expanded coverage and cost control will be paralyzing. As discussed in chapter 2, American political culture tends toward trickle-down absolutism. There can be only one dominant right at a time, so a universal right to health care is seen to threaten the right to life of vulnerable members of our society. This way of framing the rights tradeoff, of course, ignores the people who die prematurely due to lack of insurance coverage, a number that is estimated to run into the tens of thousands each year.[21] People dying from undiagnosed ailments or poorly managed chronic disease do not make the headlines. They are not on the radar of prolife activists whose attention at life's end is concentrated on one particular setting—the physician-patient encounter in a hospital where acute care might save a patient's life. The lack of similar moral urgency for community wellness, prevention, and cost-effective care contributes to the cultural reality that some economically disadvantaged patients have experienced the morbidity of untreated illness most of their days or do not trust a health care system to which they have only tenuous access. As their lives wane, these marginalized patients may experience a newfound commitment from hospitals geared to provide lifesaving care and from a culture demanding aggressive heroic medicine in the operating room and intensive-care unit. Although Americans all potentially face this scene, it exercises such a profound hold over the moral imagination that it distracts us from the fuller meanings of dignity and stewardship in religious traditions.

Human dignity is a complex value. In Jewish and Christian traditions, the dignity that God confers on human beings is absolute. Simultaneously, however, other moral considerations cluster around it, including responsibility, vulnerability, flourishing, mutuality. Conservatives tend to place personal responsibility at the center of health care justice, with social obligations to the most vulnerable as an essential guarantee of a family-centric ethics of life. Liberals typically locate health care justice in the mutuality of health need and the shared responsibility for meeting it over the entire course of a flourishing life. Putting these two ethics into conversation, the blessings of life and the blessings of living well are seen as integrally connected in a fuller accounting of human dignity and the reverence and respect it commands.

Also closely related to dignity is stewardship. Personal stewardship of physical and mental health is one of the moral strings attached to God's gift of life, no matter how spiritualized a view of the healing powers of faith a congregation might take. At the same time, social stewardship of health care resources is called for to ensure the community's ability to protect and promote people's dignity. Dignity is not a free pass that excuses all personal responsibility for attending to one's health. Dignity is not a switch that turns on only in health care crisis when life's survival is at stake. The absolutism of rights politics in America makes the public arena the wrong place to sort through the moral wisdom embedded in conservative and liberal religious visions of human dignity and its stewardship. Congregations are more promising spaces for these difficult conversations because congregations perform their shared responsibilities for healing primarily through abundant sharing in blessing, relationship, well-being, and hope.

Increasingly, Americans see hospice as an acceptable final stop before the final rest. Palliative medicine has made inroads into hospital routines, but the finality of death consigns these care options to the category of last resort. A culture of faith in the next miracle cure and a culture of silence around dying as intrinsic to human life and inescapable in health care leave Americans unprepared to speak with family, friends, congregants, or community members about their desires for health and healing as life's end nears. In the words of the Evangelical Lutheran Church in America's statement on "Caring for Health: Our Shared Endeavor," "Such cultural attitudes lead to increasing reliance upon expensive curative medicine without significantly extending life span or improving quality of life. They also too often leave individuals to struggle alone with the ethical challenges raised by advances in medicine."[22]

This moral isolation is exacerbated by the imbalance between dignity and stewardship in the American way of dying. Because protecting dignity looms so large in our bioethical and medical imagination, the default position is to "do everything possible" for a loved one. The issue of stewardship rarely arises. Out of fear of indignity, it is hard to ask two questions: How do patients want to steward their health as life declines? What responsibilities do they see themselves having for stewarding shared health care resources? Families and fellow congregants should be asking one another these questions. The difficulty is that stewardship means working within limits. Acknowledging limits in care for the dying conflicts with our refusal to recognize the limits of life. When political grenades like the "death panel scare" explode into public debates, cultural support for discussing the limits we are willing to live with fades even more. Stewardship becomes a cultural taboo.[23]

Such scare tactics should not be allowed to stand past the weekend following Muslim Friday prayers, Saturday Sabbath worship, and Sunday church services. Religious congregations are not the arbiters of American politics, of course. Instead they are communities, places where a shared faith in common worship can help supplant the culture of faith in the next technological miracle. When congregants are asked to hold the sick in their prayers, the image should be of a community holding out wholeness to a person in the form of emotional, mental, and spiritual support even as physical health wanes. The practice of remembering sick and departed members should be a self-reflective way both to acknowledge the blessings of wholeness in one's present life and to seek the strength to accept an evolving wholeness as one's life moves toward its end. These weekly practices can set the stage for the conversations about dying well that are so hard even in congregations where the profession of human finitude is as frequent as the delight in life. If acted upon outside of worship, these ritual practices can enter into the mercies of health care, too.

Congregations are not the only sites for the cultural work of balancing the value tensions involved in implementing the individual and employer mandates, shifting US health care away from acute medicine toward community-based care, and learning to speak together about dying well. Given the common religious commitments to healing as a shared responsibility, however, congregations should lead the way in acting on the mercies of health care. Mercy runs through all three value tensions. These mercies include ensuring the ACA's mandates remain affordable; supporting one another's healthy habits to lower the system's costs; making community health centers the primary care home for uninsured patients; accompanying newly insured Americans on their journeys; being responsive to the health needs and assets in underserved communities; supporting ailing neighbors in their homes, especially after release from the hospital; bringing emotional, spiritual, and mental healing to the elderly and terminally ill; recognizing the limits of our lives and consoling family and friends by setting clear priorities and limits as we steward the health remaining to us, always with an eye to stewarding the social good of US health care.

Putting the mercies of health care first can open up the national reform debate, and it can motivate wider action on behalf of healthier communities. Mercy is a meeting place. Mercy is a response that summons forth further responses. This kind of moral exchange—responding to one another's health needs and one another's health care values—can shift public debates outside the familiar conceptions of health care justice. Currently, Americans approach health care justice through the three common languages of health care as a private benefit, private choice, and public right. Instead, US health care is a social good, however incomplete the social coordination has been so far. The more that rights take center stage in the reform debate, the more that the brittleness of rights politics leaves Americans in warring camps, unwilling to engage over how to balance health care values and, more importantly, how to build up the nation's capacities for community-based care as essential to good health and social stewardship. A new civic space for hearing out and acting on the full range of health care values will require more than big religious provider organizations sharing their values. It will take religious congregations and interfaith coalitions engaging in moral dialogue and community action, translating the traditional shared responsibilities for healing into new words and deeds for today.

NOTES

1. Kaiser Family Foundation, *Health Care Costs*, 25.
2. Congressional Budget Office, *CBO's 2011 Long-Term Budget Outlook*, 35. For evidence that the recent slowdown in health care spending growth may persist because of structural changes, see Cutler and Sahni, "If Slow Rate of Health Care Spending Persists."
3. Baicker and Finkelstein, "The Effects of Medicaid Coverage." For full results, see Finkelstein et al., "The Oregon Health Insurance Experiment."
4. Zoloth, *Health Care and the Ethics of Encounter*, 29–30.
5. Ibid., 36–47.
6. Kolata, "Panel Urges Mammograms at 50"; Harris, "U.S. Panel Says No to Prostate Screening."
7. Pear, "Obama Panel to Curb Medicare Finds Foes."
8. Kaiser Family Foundation, *Health Care Costs*, 25–26.
9. Ebeler et al., "Independent Payment Advisory Board," 10.
10. Uninsured Americans, without a waiver for financial hardship or a variety of other exceptions, must obtain health coverage or face annual fines up to the greater of $695 per person ($2,085 per family) or 2.5 percent of household income. Employers with more than fifty full-time workers must either pay $2,000 per worker (excluding the first thirty employees) if they offer no coverage or pay $3,000 per worker who obtains insurance through a state insurance exchange if they offer coverage. See Kaiser Family Foundation, "Summary of the Affordable Care Act."

11. Ebeler et al., "Independent Payment Advisory Board," 5–9.

12. Mechanic et al., "The New Era of Payment Reform," 2335.

13. Ibid., 2336–38.

14. Ibid., 2339.

15. Zoloth, *Health Care and the Ethics of Encounter*, 29–32.

16. Churchill, *Rationing Health Care in America*, 99.

17. Mackler notes that mercy is more central to Catholic (and I would add other Christian) health care ethics than it is to Jewish ethics where justice predominates. Yet the rabbis stressed that God's right hand of mercy is stronger than the left hand of justice. See Mackler, *Introduction to Jewish and Catholic Bioethics*, 201.

18. Hamilton, "Continue to Care."

19. Memphis, Tennessee, has been a hotbed for health ministries. See Hotz and Mathews, *Dust and Breath*, on the Church Health Center. See Smietana, "The Power of Partnership" on Methodist Le Bonheur. Gary Gunderson has discussed congregational contributions to health ministry in many books, including Gunderson and Pray, *Leading Causes of Life*.

20. Riley and Lubitz, "Long-Term Trends in Medicare Payments in the Last Year of Life," 571.

21. The Institute of American Medicine estimated that in 2001 over eighteen thousand Americans died from poorly treated chronic disease because they lacked secure health coverage (*Care without Coverage*). A later study using a different methodology raised this figure to over forty-four thousand annual deaths in 2006 (Wilper et al., "Health Insurance and Mortality in US Adults").

22. Evangelical Lutheran Church in America, "Caring for Health," 1.

23. Pear, "U.S. Alters Rule on Paying for End-of-Life Planning."

Bibliography

Altman, Stuart H., Uwe E. Reinhardt, and Alexandra E. Shields, eds. *The Future of the U.S. Healthcare System: Who Will Care for the Poor and Uninsured?* Chicago, IL: Health Administration Press; and Waltham, MA: Council on the Economic Impact of Health System Change, 1998.

American Hospital Association. "Aggregate Hospital Payment-to-Cost Ratios for Private Payers, Medicare and Medicaid, 1989–2009." www.aha.org/research/reports/tw/chartbook/2011/table4-4.pdf (accessed Mar. 30, 2012).

———. "Results of the 2009 Schedule H Project," Jan. 2012. www.aha.org/research/policy/finfactsheets.shtml (accessed Sept. 27, 2012).

Arbuckle, Gerald A. *Healthcare Ministry: Refounding the Mission in Tumultuous Times.* Collegeville, MN: Liturgical Press, 2000.

Arrow, Kenneth J. "Uncertainty and the Welfare Economics of Medical Care." *The American Economic Review* 53, no. 5 (1963): 941–73.

Association of American Medical Colleges. "Table 6: Revenues Supporting Programs and Activities at All 126 Fully Accredited U.S. Medical Schools FY2008–FY2010." https://www.aamc.org/data/finance/2010tables/ (accessed Dec. 12, 2013).

Audi, Robert, and Nicholas Wolterstorff. *Religion in the Public Square: The Place of Religious Convictions in Political Debate.* Lanham, MD: Rowman and Littlefield, 1996.

Ayanian, John Z., and Philip J. Van der Wees. "Tackling Rising Health Care Costs in Massachusetts." *New England Journal of Medicine* 367 (Aug. 30, 2012): 790–93.

Baicker, Katherine, and Amy Finkelstein. "The Effects of Medicaid Coverage—Learning from the Oregon Medicaid Experiment." *New England Journal of Medicine* 365 (Aug. 25, 2011): 683–85.

Barr, Donald A. *Introduction to U.S. Health Policy: The Organizing, Financing, and Delivery of Health Care in America*, 3d. ed. Baltimore, MD: Johns Hopkins University Press, 2007.

Bazzoli, Gloria J., Anneliese Gerland, and Jessica May. "Trends: Construction Activity in U.S. Hospitals." *Health Affairs* 25, no. 3 (2006): 783–91.

Beauchamp, Dan. *Health Care Reform and the Battle for the Body Politic.* Philadelphia: Temple University Press, 1994.

Becker, Cinda. "Charity with an Arm Twist." *Modern Healthcare* 36, no. 37 (2006): 6–16.

Benne, Robert. *The Paradoxical Vision: A Public Theology for the Twenty-First Century*. Minneapolis, MN: Fortress Press, 1995.

Bernardin, Joseph. "A Consistent Ethic of Life: An American-Catholic Dialogue." In *Consistent Ethic of Life*. Kansas City, MO: Sheed and Ward, 1988.

Brill, Steven. "Bitter Pill." *Time* 181, no. 8 (Mar. 4, 2013): 16–55.

Brown, Lawrence D. "Health Reform in America: The Mystery of the Missing Moral Momentum." *Conservative Judaism* 51, no. 4 (1999): 103–11.

Butler, Stuart. "A New Policy Framework for Health Care Markets." *Health Affairs* 23, no. 2 (2004): 22–24.

Cahill, Lisa Sowle. *Theological Bioethics: Participation, Justice, Change*. Washington, DC: Georgetown University Press, 2005.

Callahan, Daniel. "Medicine and the Market: A Research Agenda." *Journal of Medicine and Philosophy* 24, no. 3 (1999): 224–42.

Cannon, Michael F., and Michael D. Tanner. *Healthy Competition: What's Holding Back Health Care and How to Free It*, 2d. ed. Washington, DC: Cato Institute, 2007.

Carlson, Joe, and Vince Galloro. "Big Dividends." *Modern Healthcare* 40, no. 3 (2010): 18–28.

Casalino, Lawrence P., Kelly J. Devers, and Linda R. Brewster. "Focused Factories: Physician-Owned Specialty Facilities." *Health Affairs* 22, no. 6 (2003): 56–67.

Catholic Health Association (with VHA Inc.). *A Guide for Planning and Reporting Community Benefit*. St. Louis, MO: Catholic Health Association, 2006.

Centers for Disease Control. "Chronic Diseases: The Power to Prevent, the Call to Control: At a Glance 2009." Last modified Dec. 17, 2009. www.cdc.gov/chronicdisease/resources/publications/AAG/chronic.htm.

Chapman, Audrey R. "Health Care Reform: The Potential Contributions of a Faith-Based Approach." *Journal of the Society of Christian Ethics* 28, no. 2 (2008): 205–21.

Churchill, Larry R. *Rationing Health Care in America: Perceptions and Principles of Justice*. Notre Dame, IN: University of Notre Dame Press, 1987.

Cochran, Clarke E. "Institutional Identity; Sacramental Potential: Catholic Healthcare at Century's End." *Christian Bioethics* 5, no. 1 (1999): 26–43.

Colombo, John D. "The Failure of Community Benefit." *Health Matrix: Journal of Law-Medicine* 15, no. 29 (2005): 29–65.

Congressional Budget Office. *CBO's 2011 Long-Term Budget Outlook*, June 2011. www.cbo.gov/publication/41486 (accessed Dec. 29, 2012).

———. "Estimates for the Insurance Coverage Provisions of the Affordable Care Act Updated for the Recent Supreme Court Decision," July 2012. www.cbo.gov/publication/43472 (accessed Sept. 12, 2012).

Cooper, Helene. "Nuns Back Bill amid Broad Rift over Whether It Limits Abortion Enough." *New York Times*, Mar. 20, 2010, A10.

Cooper, Helene, and Laurie Goodstein. "Rule Shift on Birth Control Is Concession to Obama Allies." *New York Times*, Feb. 2, 2012, A1.

Craig, David M. "Everyone at the Table: Religious Activism and Health Care Reform in Massachusetts." *Journal of Religious Ethics* 40, no. 2 (2012): 336–59.

———. "Religious Health Care as Community Benefit: Social Contract, Common Good, or Covenant?" *Kennedy Institute of Ethics Journal* 18, no. 4 (2008): 301–30.

Cram, Peter, Gary E. Rosenthal, and Mary S. Vaughan-Sarrazin. "Cardiac Revascularization in Specialty and General Hospitals." *New England Journal of Medicine* 352, no. 14 (Apr. 7, 2005): 1454–62.

Cunningham, Peter. "Nonurgent Use of Emergency Departments." Statement Before the U.S. Senate Committee on Health, Education, Labor, and Pensions Committee, Subcommittee on Primary Health and Aging, May 11, 2011.

Curran, Charles E. "The Catholic Identity of Catholic Institutions." *Theological Studies* 58, no. 1 (1997): 90–108.

Cutler, David, and Nikhil R. Sahni. "If Slow Rate of Health Care Spending Persists, Then Projections May Be Off by $770 Billion." *Health Affairs* 32, no. 5 (2013): 841–50.

Daniels, Norman. *Just Health Care*. Cambridge, MA: Cambridge University Press, 1985.

———. *Just Health: Meeting Health Needs Fairly*. Cambridge, MA: Cambridge University Press, 2007.

Daniels, Norman, Bruce P. Kennedy, and Ichiro Kawachi. "Justice, Health and Health Policy." In Danis, Clancy, and Churchill, *Ethical Dimensions of Health Policy*, 19–47.

Danis, Marion, Carolyn Clancy, and Larry R. Churchill, eds. *Ethical Dimensions of Health Policy*. New York: Oxford University Press, 2002.

DeBoer, Michael J. "Religious Hospitals and the Federal Community Benefit Standard: Counting Religious Purpose as a Tax-Exemption Factor for Hospitals." *Seton Hall Law Review* 42, no. 4 (2012): 1549–1634.

DiNardo, Daniel D. "Letter on Conscience Protection." Washington, DC: U.S. Conference of Catholic Bishops, Aug. 3, 2012. www.usccb.org/issues-and-action/religious -liberty/conscience-protection/upload/Cardinal-DiNardo-s-August-2012-Letter-to -Congress-Regarding-Conscience-Protection.pdf (accessed Nov. 13, 2012).

Dolan, Jay P. "Social Catholicism." In *Making the Nonprofit Sector in the United States*, edited by David C. Hammack, 189–202. Bloomington: Indiana University Press, 1998.

Dorff, Elliot N. "Am I My Brother's Keeper?: A Jewish View on the Distribution of Health Care." *Conservative Judaism* 51, no. 4 (1999): 13–30.

———. "Assisted Death: A Jewish Perspective." In Hamel and DuBose, *Must We Suffer Our Way to Death?*, 141–73.

———. *Love Your Neighbor and Yourself: A Jewish Approach to Modern Personal Ethics*. Philadelphia: Jewish Publication Society, 2006.

———. *Matters of Life and Death: A Jewish Approach to Modern Medical Ethics*. Philadelphia: Jewish Publication Society, 1998.

Dorff, Elliot N., and Louis E. Newman, eds. *Contemporary Jewish Ethics and Morality: A Reader*. Oxford: Oxford University Press, 1995.

Dorsey, E. Ray, et al. "Funding of U.S. Biomedical Research, 2003–2008." *The Journal of the American Medical Association* 303, no. 2 (2010): 137–43.

Dougherty, Charles J. *Back to Reform: Values, Markets, and the Health Care System.* New York: Oxford University Press, 1996.

Dranove, David, and Michael L. Millenson. "Medical Bankruptcy: Myth Versus Fact." *Health Affairs* 25 (2006): w74–w83. http://content.healthaffairs.org/content/25/2/w74.full.pdf+html (accessed Feb. 10, 2012).

Dubler, Nancy Neveloff. "Introduction." *Conservative Judaism* 51, no. 4 (1999): 6–12.

Ebeler, Jack, Tricia Neuman, and Juliette Cubanski, "The Independent Payment Advisory Board: A New Approach to Controlling Medicare Spending." Menlo Park, CA: Kaiser Family Foundation Program on Medicaid Policy, April 2011. www.kff.org/medicare/upload/8150.pdf (accessed Dec. 29, 2012).

Elshtain, Jean Bethke. "Health Care Reform and Finitude." *Conservative Judaism* 51, no. 4 (1999): 65–71.

Families USA. *Hidden Health Tax: Americans Pay a Premium.* Washington, DC: Families USA: 2009. http://familiesusa2.org/assets/pdfs/hidden-health-tax.pdf (accessed Feb. 10, 2012).

Finkelstein, Amy. "The Aggregate Effects of Health Insurance: Evidence from the Introduction of Medicare." NBER working paper 11619. Cambridge, MA: National Bureau of Economic Research, 2005.

Finkelstein, Amy, and Robin McKnight. "What Did Medicare Do (And Was It Worth It)?" NBER working paper 11609. Cambridge, MA: National Bureau of Economic Research, 2005.

Finkelstein, Amy, et al. "The Oregon Health Insurance Experiment: Evidence from the First Year." NBER working paper 17190. Cambridge, MA: National Bureau of Economic Research, July 2011.

Frakt, Austin B. "How Much Do Hospitals Cost Shift? A Review of the Evidence." *The Milbank Quarterly* 89, no. 1 (2011): 90–130.

Fried, Charles. Testimony to the Senate Committee on Judiciary Hearing on the "Constitutionality of the Affordable Care Act," Feb. 2, 2011. www.judiciary.senate.gov/pdf/11-02-02%20Fried%20Testimony.pdf (accessed Feb. 10, 2012).

George, Francis. "Universal Health Care." Washington, DC: U.S. Conference of Catholic Bishops, Mar. 23, 2010. http://old.usccb.org/healthcare/cardinal-george-health care-statement.pdf (accessed Nov. 13, 2012).

Ginzberg, Eli. "Health-Care Policy in the United States in the 20th Century." In Danis, Clancy, and Churchill, *Ethical Dimensions of Health Policy*, 65–76.

Goldhill, David. "The Health Benefits That Cut Your Pay." *New York Times*, Feb. 17, 2013, SR6–7.

Goodman, John C. "Designing Health Insurance for the Information Age." In Herzlinger, *Consumer-Driven Health Care*, 224–41.

Grassley, Charles. "IRS Report Shows Non-Profit Hospitals Often Provide Little Charity Care." Press release, US Senator Charles Grassley, July 19, 2007. http://grass

ley.senate.gov/news/Article.cfm?customel_dataPageID _1502 = 8990 (accessed Oct. 18, 2008).

Green, Ronald M. "Health Care and Justice in Contract Theory Perspective." In *Ethics and Health Policy*, edited by Robert M. Veatch and Roy Branson, 111–26. Cambridge, MA: Ballinger, 1976.

———. "The Priority of Health Care." *The Journal of Medicine and Philosophy* 8 (1983): 373–80.

Greenwald, Leslie, et al. "Specialty Versus Community Hospitals: Referrals, Quality, and Community Benefits." *Health Affairs* 25, no. 1 (2006): 106–18.

Gruber, Jonathan. "The Role of Consumer Copayments for Health Care: Lessons from the RAND Health Insurance Experiment and Beyond." Menlo Park, CA: Kaiser Family Foundation, Oct. 2006. www.kff.org/insurance/7566.cfm (accessed June 27, 2007).

Gunderson, Gary, and Larry M. Pray. *Leading Causes of Life: Five Fundamentals to Change the Way You Live Your Life*. Nashville, TN: Abingdon, 2009.

Guterman, Stuart. "Specialty Hospitals: A Problem or a Symptom?" *Health Affairs* 25, no. 1 (2006): 95–105.

Gutmann, Amy, and Dennis Thompson. "Just Deliberation about Health Care." In Danis, Clancy, and Churchill, *Ethical Dimensions of Health Policy*, 77–94.

Hadley, Jack, John Holahan, Teresa Coughlin, and Dawn Miller. "Covering the Uninsured in 2008: Current Costs, Sources of Payment, and Incremental Costs." *Health Affairs* 27, no. 5 (2008): w399–w415. http://content.healthaffairs.org/content/27/5/w399.full.pdf + html (accessed June 21, 2012).

Hamel, Ronald P., and Edwin R. DuBose, eds. *Must We Suffer Our Way to Death? Cultural and Theological Perspectives on Death by Choice*. Dallas: Southern Methodist University Press, 1996.

Hamilton, Hurmon E., Jr. "A Call to Action!" *CommonHealth*, July 16, 2008. For all of Hamilton's posts, see WBUR's blog *CommonHealth: Reform and Reality* at http://archives.commonhealth.wbur.org// (accessed Nov. 11, 2010).

———. "Come Now, and Let Us Reason Together." *CommonHealth*, May 27, 2008.

———. "Continue to Care: A Valentine's Day Affirmation." *CommonHealth*, Jan. 31, 2008.

———. "A Dying Hope on Easter Sunday Morning." *CommonHealth*, Apr. 8, 2007.

———. "Give to Caesar, What Is Caesar's!" *CommonHealth*, Sept. 3, 2008.

———. "Health Care Reform: Where Do We Go from Here?" *CommonHealth*, Feb. 28, 2007.

———. "Responding to the Signs of the Times with Sound Judgement and Resounding Justice!" *CommonHealth*, Feb. 18, 2009.

———. "Successful Implementation Requires Real Outreach and Enrollment." *CommonHealth*, May 9, 2007.

———. "This Is the Day the LORD Has Made; Let Us Rejoice and Be Glad in It." *CommonHealth*, June 4, 2007.

————. "Truly Fair and Reasonable." *CommonHealth*, July 17, 2007.

————. "Walking through the Valley of the Shadow of Death." *CommonHealth*, July 28, 2009.

————. "What Is the Character of Our Commonwealth?" *CommonHealth*, May 19, 2009.

————. "Why Outreach and Enrollment Matters." *CommonHealth*, Apr. 22, 2008.

Hanson, Jack. "Are We Getting Our Money's Worth? Charity Care, Community Benefits, and Tax Exemption at Nonprofit Hospitals." *Loyola Consumer Law Review* 17 (2005): 395–417.

Harris, Gardiner. "Federal Research Center Will Help Develop Medicines." *New York Times*, Jan. 23, 2011, A1.

————. "U.S. Panel Says No to Prostate Screening for Healthy Men." *New York Times*, Nov. 7, 2011, A1.

Hauerwas, Stanley. "Christian Critique of Christian America." In *The Hauerwas Reader*, edited by John Berkman and Michael Cartwright, 459–80. Durham, NC: Duke University Press, 2001.

Hawkins, Jessica L. "Separating Fact from Fiction: Mandated Insurance Coverage of Infertility Treatments." *Washington University Journal of Law and Policy* 23 (2007): 203–27.

Helms, Robert B. "Tax Policy and the History of the Health Insurance Industry." In *Using Taxes to Reform Health Insurance: Pitfalls and Promises*, edited by Henry J. Aaron and Leonard E. Burman, 13–35. Washington, DC: Brookings Institution Press, 2008.

Henderson, Thomas. *Medicaid Direct and Indirect Graduate Medical Education Payments: A 50-State Survey 2010*. Washington, DC: Association of American Medical Colleges, 2010. https://members.aamc.org/eweb/DynamicPage.aspx?webcode = PubSearch Results (accessed May 24, 2012).

Herzlinger, Regina E. "Diagnosis: What, Precisely, Is Wrong with the American Health-System." *National Review*, May 25, 2009: 26–32.

————. *Market-Driven Health Care: Who Wins, Who Loses in the Transformation of America's Largest Service Industry*. Reading, MA: Addison-Wesley, 1997.

————. "Why We Need Consumer-Driven Health Care." In Herzlinger, *Consumer-Driven Health Care*, 1–197.

Herzlinger, Regina E., ed. *Consumer-Driven Health Care: Implications for Providers, Payers, and Policymakers*. San Francisco: Jossey-Bass, 2004.

Himmelstein, David U., Deborah Thorne, Elizabeth Warren, and Steffie Woolhandler. "Medical Bankruptcy in the United States, 2007: Results of a National Study." *The American Journal of Medicine* 20, no. 10 (2009): 1–6.

Hoffman, Catherine. *National Health Insurance: A Brief History of Reform Efforts in the U.S.* Washington, DC: Kaiser Family Foundation, 2009. http://kaiserfamilyfoundation.files.wordpress.com/2013/01/7871.pdf (accessed May 15, 2012).

Holahan, John, and Allison Cook. "The U.S. Economy and Changes in Health Insurance Coverage, 2000–2006." *Health Affairs* 27, no. 2 (2008): w135–w144. http://content.healthaffairs.org/cgi/content/full/27/2/w135 (accessed Mar. 10, 2008).

Hollenbach, David. *The Common Good and Christian Ethics.* Cambridge, MA: Cambridge University Press, 2002.

Hotz, Kendra G., and Mathew T. Matthews. *Dust and Breath: Faith, Health, and Why the Church Should Care about Both.* Grand Rapids, MI: Eerdmans, 2012.

Hunter, James Davison. *Culture Wars: The Struggle to Define America.* New York: Basic Books, 1992.

Iglehart, John K. "Health Centers Fill Critical Gap, Enjoy Support." *Health Affairs* 29, no. 3 (2010): 343–45.

———. "Health Care USA: Economic Product or Social Good?" *British Medical Journal* 290 (1985): 257–58.

Institute of Medicine. *America's Uninsured Crisis: Consequences for Health and Health Care.* Washington, DC: National Academies Press, 2009.

———. *Care without Coverage, Too Little, Too Late.* Washington, DC: National Academies Press, 2002.

Jacobs, Jill. *There Shall Be No Needy: Pursuing Social Justice through Jewish Law and Tradition.* Woodstock, VT: Jewish Lights Publishing, 2010.

Japsen, Bruce. "Provena Files Appeal over Tax: Cites 'Errors' in State Tally of Charity Care." *Chicago Tribune,* Oct. 27, 2006.

Joint Committee on Taxation. "Background Materials for Senate Committee on Finance Roundtable on Health Care Financing." Senate Committee on Finance, May 12, 2009. http://finance.senate.gov/JCT.pdf (accessed Feb. 6, 2012).

Kaiser Commission on Medicaid and the Uninsured. "Five Key Questions about Medicaid and Its Role in State/Federal Budgets and Health Reform." Washington, DC: Kaiser Family Foundation, May 2012. http://kaiserfamilyfoundation.files.wordpress.com/2013/01/8139-02.pdf (accessed June 19, 2012).

Kaiser Family Foundation. *Employer Health Benefits 2012.* Menlo Park, CA: Kaiser Family Foundation, Sept. 11, 2012. http://kff.org/private-insurance/report/employer-health-benefits-2012-annual-survey/ (accessed Oct. 9, 2012).

———. "Federal Medicaid Disproportionate Share (DSH) Allotments." http://kff.org/medicaid/state-indicator/federal-dsh-allotments/ (accessed May 10, 2012).

———. *Health Care Costs: A Primer: Key Information on Health Care Costs and Their Impact.* Menlo Park, CA: Kaiser Family Foundation, 2012. http://kaiserfamilyfoundation.files.wordpress.com/2013/01/7670-03.pdf (accessed Dec. 29, 2012).

———. "Health Insurance Coverage of the Nonelderly Population, 2011." http://kff.org/slideshow/health-insurance-coverage-in-america-2011/ (accessed Jan. 15, 2013).

———. "Health Insurance Coverage of the Total Population, 2011." http://kff.org/other/state-indicator/total-population (accessed Oct. 26, 2012).

———. "Proposed Changes to Medicare in the 'Path to Prosperity.'" Menlo Park, CA: Kaiser Family Foundation, April 2011. http://kaiserfamilyfoundation.files.wordpress.com/2013/04/8179.pdf (accessed Mar. 31, 2013).

———. "Summary of the Affordable Care Act." Last modified April 23, 2013. http://
kaiserfamilyfoundation.files.wordpress.com/2011/04/8061-021.pdf.

———. "Tax Subsidies for Health Insurance: An Issue Brief." Menlo Park, CA: Kaiser
Family Foundation, 2008. http://kaiserfamilyfoundation.files.wordpress.com/2013/
01/7779.pdf (accessed June 25, 2011).

———. "The Uninsured and the Difference Health Insurance Makes," Sept. 1, 2012.
http://kff.org/uninsured/fact-sheet/the-uninsured-and-the-difference-health-insur
ance/ (accessed Jan. 15, 2013).

———. "United States: Federally Qualified Health Centers, 2010 Data." www.state
healthfacts.org/profileind.jsp?cat = 8&sub = 99&rgn = 1 (accessed Apr. 20, 2012).

Kaiser Family Foundation Program on Medicaid Policy. "Independent Payment Advisory Board: A New Approach to Controlling Medicare Spending." Menlo Park, CA:
Kaiser Family Foundation, April 2011. http://kaiserfamilyfoundation.files.wordpress
.com/2013/01/8150.pdf (accessed Dec. 29, 2012).

Kaiser Health News. "Transcript: GOP Candidates Squabble over Health Care during
Tampa Debate," Sept. 13, 2011. www.kaiserhealthnews.org/Stories/2011/September
/13/transcript-gop-debate-health-care-issues.aspx (accessed Nov. 10, 2011).

Katz, Robert A. "Paging Dr. Shylock! Jewish Hospitals and the Prudent Re-investment
of Jewish Philanthropy." In *Giving: For the Love of God*, edited by David H. Smith,
162–84. Bloomington: Indiana University Press.

Kauffman, Christopher J. *Ministry and Meaning: A Religious History of Catholic Health
Care in the United States*. New York: Crossroad, 1995.

Kaveny, M. Cathleen. "Commodifying the Polyvalent Good of Health Care." *Journal
of Medicine and Philosophy* 24, no. 3 (1999): 207–23.

Keehan, Carol. "The Tax-Exempt Sector." Testimony Before the Full Committee of the
House Committee on Ways and Means, May 26, 2005. http://waysandmeans.house
.gov/hearings.asp?formmode = view&id = 2718 (accessed Oct. 18, 2008).

Keehan, Sean P., et al. "National Health Spending Projections through 2020: Economic
Recovery and Reform Drive Faster Spending Growth." *Health Affairs* 30, no. 8
(2011): 1594–1605.

King, Martin Luther, Jr. *A Testament of Hope: The Essential Writings and Speeches of
Martin Luther King, Jr.*, edited by James M. Washington. San Francisco: Harper-
Collins, 1991.

Kleinke, J. D. "The Conservative Case for Obamacare." *New York Times*, Sept. 30,
2012, SR4.

Kolata, Gina. "Panel Urges Mammograms at 50, Not 40." *New York Times*, Nov. 17,
2009, A1.

Kraut, Alan M., and Deborah A. Kraut. *Covenant of Care: Newark Beth Israel and the
Jewish Hospital in America*. New Brunswick, NJ: Rutgers University Press, 2006.

Kronick, Richard. "Valuing Charity." *Journal of Health Politics, Policy, and Law* 26,
no. 5 (2001): 993–1001.

Krugman, Paul. "Health Care Realities." *New York Times*, July 31, 2009, A23.

Laird, Lance D., and Wendy Cadge. "Muslims, Medicine, and Mercy: Free Clinics in Southern California." In *Not by Faith Alone: Social Services, Social Justice, and Faith-based Organizations in the United States*, edited by Julie Adkins, Laurie Occhipinti, and Tara Heffernan, 107–28. Lanham, MD: Lexington Books, 2010.

Lalli, Frank. "A Health Insurance Detective Story." *New York Times*, Dec. 12, 2012, SR5.

Leo XIII, *Rerum novarum*. 1891. www.vatican.va/holy_father/leo_xiii/encyclicals/docu ments/hf_l-xiii_enc_15051891_rerum-novarum_en.html (accessed Oct. 11, 2012).

Long, Sharon K., Karen Stockley, and Heather Dahlen. "Massachusetts Health Reforms: Uninsurance Remains Low, Self-Reported Health Status Improves as State Prepares to Tackle Costs." *Health Affairs* 31, no. 2 (2012): 1–8.

Lovett, Stuart. "Chronic Problems, Innovative Solutions: Paving the Way to the Focused Factory." In Herzlinger, *Consumer-Driven Health Care*, 635–42.

Mackler, Aaron L. *Introduction to Jewish and Catholic Bioethics: A Comparative Analysis*. Washington, DC: Georgetown University Press, 2003.

Madigan, Lisa. "Madigan Proposes Two Bills to Hold Hospitals Accountable for Charity Care, Stop Unfair Billing and Collection Practices." Press release, Illinois Attorney General's Office, Jan. 23, 2006. www.illinoisattorneygeneral.gov/pressroom/2006 _01/20060123.html (accessed 18 October 2008).

Maritain, Jacques. *The Person and the Common Good*, translated by John J. Fitzgerald. South Bend, IN: University of Notre Dame, 1966.

Martin, Anne B., David Lassman, Benjamin Washington, and Aaron Catlin. "Growth in US Health Spending Remained Slow in 2010." *Health Affairs* 31, no. 1 (2012): 208–19.

Massachusetts Division of Health Care Finance and Policy. "Health Insurance Coverage in Massachusetts," 2010. www.mass.gov/eohhs/docs/dhcfp/r/pubs/10/mhis-report -12-2010.pdf (accessed Oct. 26, 2012).

———. "Massachusetts Employer Survey 2010." www.mass.gov/eohhs/docs/dhcfp/r/ pubs/11/mes-results-2010.pdf (accessed Oct. 26, 2012).

May, William F. "The Burned." Chap. 2, *The Patient's Ordeal*, 15–35. Bloomington: Indiana University Press, 1994.

———. "Code, Covenant, Contract, or Philanthropy." *Hastings Center Report* 5 (Dec. 1975): 29–38.

———. *The Physician's Covenant: Images of the Healer in Medical Ethics*. Philadelphia: Westminster Press, 1983.

———. *Testing the Medical Covenant: Active Euthanasia and Health Care Reform*. Grand Rapids, MI: Eerdmans, 1996.

McCormick, Richard A. "The Catholic Hospital: Mission Impossible?" *Origins* 24 (March 1995): 648–53.

McDonough, Mary J. *Can a Health Care Market Be Moral? A Catholic Vision*. Washington, DC: Georgetown University Press, 2007.

McKethan, Aaron, Nadia Nguyen, Benjamin E. Sasse, and S. Lawrence Kocot. "Reforming the Medicaid Disproportionate-Share Hospital Program." *Health Affairs* 28, no. 5 (2009): w926–36. http://content.healthaffairs.org/content/28/5/w926.full (accessed Apr. 26, 2012).

Mechanic, Robert E., Stuart H. Altman, and John E. McDonough. "The New Era of Payment Reform, Spending Targets, and Cost Containment in Massachusetts: Early Lessons for the Nation." *Health Affairs* 31, no. 10 (2012): 2334–42.

Medicare Payment Advisory Commission. *Aligning Incentives in Medicare.* Washington, DC: Medpac, 2010. www.medpac.gov/documents/jun10_entirereport.pdf (accessed May 24, 2012).

———. *Physician-Owned Specialty Hospitals Revisited.* Washington, DC: Medpac, 2006. www.medpac.gov/documents/Aug06_specialtyhospital_mandated_report.pdf (accessed Oct. 18, 2012).

Miller, Tom. "Massachusetts: More Mirage Than Miracle." *Health Affairs* 25, no. 6 (2006): w450–w452. http://content.healthaffairs.org/content/25/6/w450.full (accessed June 26, 2007).

Moffit, Robert Emmett. "Personal Freedom and Responsibility: The Ethical Foundations of a Market-Based Health Care Reform." *Journal of Medicine and Philosophy* 19, no. 5 (1994): 471–81.

Moses, Hamilton, and Joseph B. Martin. "Biomedical Research and Health Advances." *New England Journal of Medicine* 364 (Feb. 10, 2011): 567–71.

Musgrave, Frank W. *The Economics of U.S. Health Policy: The Role of Market Forces.* Armonk, NY: M.E. Sharpe, 2006.

National Association of Community Health Centers. "Community Health Centers: The Return on Investment." Fact sheet, November 2010. www.nachc.com/client/documents/CHCs%20ROI%20final%2011%2015%20v.pdf (accessed Apr. 20, 2012).

Nguyen, Nguyen Xuan, and Steven H. Sheingold. "Indirect Medical Education and Disproportionate Share Adjustments to Medicare Inpatient Payment Rates." *Medicare & Medicaid Research Review* 1, no. 4 (2011): E1–E18.

Nicholson, Sean, Mark V. Pauly, Lawton R. Burns, Agnieshka Baumritter, and David A. Asch. "Measuring Community Benefits Provided by For-Profit and Nonprofit Hospitals." *Health Affairs* 19, no. 6 (2000): 168–77.

Organisation for Economic Co-Operation and Development. "Total Health Expenditures as Percent of Gross Domestic Product." Last modified Oct. 11, 2013. http://www.oecdilibrary.org/content/table/20758480-table1.

Pauly, Mark V. "Adverse Selection and Moral Hazard: Implications for Health Insurance Markets." In *Incentives and Choice in Health Care*, edited by Frank A. Sloan and Hirschel Kasper, 103–30. Cambridge, MA: MIT Press, 2008.

Pear, Robert. "Obama Panel to Curb Medicare Finds Foes in Both Parties." *New York Times*, Apr. 20, 2011, A3.

———. "U.S. Alters Rule on Paying for End-of-Life Planning." *New York Times*, Jan. 5, 2011, A15.

Pearson, Steven D., James E. Sabin, and Ezekiel J. Emanuel. *No Mission, No Margin: Health-Care Organizations and the Quest for Ethical Excellence*. New York: Oxford, 2003.

Pellegrino, Edmund D. "The Commodification of Medical and Health Care: The Moral Consequences of a Paradigm Shift from a Professional to a Market Ethic." *Journal of Medicine and Philosophy* 24, no. 3 (1999): 243–66.

Perry, Joshua E. "Physician-Owned Specialty Hospitals and the Patient Protection and Affordable Care Act: Health Care Reform at the Intersection of Law and Ethics." *American Business Law Journal* 49, no. 2 (2012): 369–417.

Powell, Walter W., and Richard Steinberg. *The Nonprofit Sector: A Research Handbook*, 2nd ed. New Haven: Yale University Press, 2006.

Principe, Kristine, E. Kathleen Adams, Jenifer Maynard, and Edmund R. Becker, "The Impact of the Individual Mandate and Internal Revenue Service Form 990 Schedule H on Community Benefits from Nonprofit Hospitals." *American Journal of Public Health* 102, no. 2 (2012): 229–37.

Quinn, Kevin. "New Directions in Medicaid Payment for Hospital Care." *Health Affairs* 27, no. 1 (2008): 269–80.

Rawls, John. "The Idea of Public Reason." Lecture 6 in *Political Liberalism*, 212–54. New York: Columbia University Press, 1993.

———. "The Idea of Public Reason Revisited." In *John Rawls: Collected Papers*, edited by Samuel Freeman, 573–622. Cambridge, MA: Harvard University Press, 1999.

Reinhardt, Uwe E. "Efficiency in Health Care." *Journal of Health Politics, Policy, and Law* 26, no. 5 (2001): 967–92.

———. "Employer-Based Health Insurance: R.I.P." In Altman, Reinhardt, and Shields, *The Future of the U.S. Healthcare System*, 325–52.

———. "Wanted: A Clearly Articulated Social Ethic for American Medicine." *Journal of the American Medical Association* 278, no. 17 (1997): 1446–47.

Rich, Eugene C., Mark Liebow, Malathi Srinivasan, David Parish, James O. Wolliscroft, Oliver Fein, and Robert Blaser. "Medicare Financing of Graduate Medical Education: Intractable Problems, Elusive Solutions." *Journal of General Internal Medicine* 17, no. 4 (2002): 283–92.

Riley, Gerald F., and James D. Lubitz, "Long-Term Trends in Medicare Payments in the Last Year of Life." *Health Services Research* 45, no. 2 (2010): 565–76.

Robert Wood Johnson Foundation. "What Are the Biggest Drivers of Cost in US Health Care?" Issue brief, July 2011. www.rwjf.org/content/dam/farm/reports/issue_briefs/2011/rwjf71331 (accessed July 10, 2012).

Robeznieks, Andis. "Fight and Flight: Some Physician Investors Getting out of Hospital Ownership While Others Stay Their Course." *Modern Healthcare* 41, no.14 (2011): 28–30.

Roob, Mitchell, and Seema Verma. "Indiana: Health Care Reform amidst Clashing Values." *Health Affairs Blog*, May 1, 2008. http://healthaffairs.org/blog/2008/05/01/indiana-health-care-reform-amidst-colliding-values/ (accessed May 18, 2010).

Rorty, Richard. "Religion as Conversation-Stopper." Chap 11, *Philosophy and Social Hope*, 168–74. London: Penguin, 1999.

Rosenthal, Meredith, and Norman Daniels, "Beyond Competition: The Normative Implications of Consumer-Driven Health Plans." *Journal of Health Politics, Policy and Law* 31, no. 3 (2006): 671–85.

Rothman, David J. "A Century of Failure: Health Care Reform in America." *Journal of Health Politics, Policy, and Law* 18, no. 2 (1993): 271–86.

Sack, Kevin. "Arizona Medicaid Cuts Seen as Signs of the Times." *New York Times*, Dec. 5, 2010, A26.

Saks, Michael. "What Do Polls Really Tell Us about the Public's View of the Affordable Care Act?" *Health Affairs Blog* Sept. 21, 2012. http://healthaffairs.org/blog/2012/09/21/what-do-polls-really-tell-us-about-the-publics-view-of-the-affordable-care-act/ (accessed Nov. 12, 2012).

Salamon, Lester M. *Partners in Public Service: Government-Nonprofit Relations in the Modern Welfare State*. Baltimore, MD: Johns Hopkins University Press, 1995.

Schlesinger, Mark, and Bradford H. Gray. "Nonprofit Organizations and Health Care: Some Paradoxes and Persistent Scrutiny." In Powell and Steinberg, *The Nonprofit Sector*, 378–414.

Shortell, Stephen M. "Bending the Cost Curve: A Critical Component of Health Care Reform." *Journal of the American Medical Association* 302, no. 11 (2009): 1223–24.

Siegel, Seymour. "A Jewish View of Economic Justice." In Dorff and Newman, *Contemporary Jewish Ethics and Morality*, 336–43.

Smietana, Bob. "The Power of Partnership." *Sojourners* 42, no. 8 (2013): 16–19.

Smith, David H., ed. *Caring Well: Religion, Narrative, and Health Care Ethics*. Louisville, KY: Westminster John Knox Press, 2000.

Starr, Paul. *The Social Transformation of American Medicine: The Rise of a Sovereign Profession and the Making of a Vast Industry*. New York: Basic Books, 1982.

Steinberg, Richard. "Economic Theories of Nonprofit Organizations." In Powell and Steinberg, *The Nonprofit Sector*, 117–39.

Steuerle, C. Eugene, and Stephanie Rennane. "Social Security and Medicare Taxes and Benefits over a Lifetime." Washington, DC: Urban Institute, 2011. www.urban.org/publications/412281.html (accessed June 22, 2011).

Stone, Robert E. "Improving Health and Reducing the Costs of Chronic Diseases." In Herzlinger, *Consumer-Driven Health Care*, 643–50.

Stout, Jeffrey. *Democracy and Tradition*. Princeton, NJ: Princeton University Press, 2004.

Tanner, Michael D. *Bad Medicine: A Guide to the Real Costs and Consequences of the New Health Care Law*. Washington, DC: Cato Institute, 2011.

Thomasson, Melissa. "The Importance of Group Coverage: How Tax Policy Shaped U.S. Health Insurance." NBER working paper 7543. Cambridge, MA: National Bureau of Economic Research, 2000.

Townes, Emilie M. *Breaking the Fine Rain of Death: African American Health Issues and a Womanist Ethic of Care*. New York: Continuum, 1998.

Truffer, Christopher J., et al. "Health Spending Projections through 2019: The Recession's Impact Continues." *Health Affairs* 29, no. 3 (2010): 522–29.

United States Catholic Bishops. *Economic Justice for All: Pastoral Letter on Catholic Social Teaching and the U.S. Economy*. Washington, DC: National Conference of Catholic Bishops, 1986. www.usccb.org/upload/economic_justice_for_all.pdf (accessed June 5, 2011).

US Census Bureau. "Table 8. Coverage by Type of Health Insurance: 2010 and 2011." www.census.gov/hhes/www/hlthins/data/incpovhlth/2011/Table8.pdf (accessed Nov. 28, 2012).

———. "Table 135. National Health Expenditures by Source of Funds: 1990 to 2009." *The 2012 Statistical Abstract*. www.census.gov/compendia/statab/2012/tables/12 s0135.pdf (accessed June 21, 2012).

US Senate Committee on Finance—Minority Staff, "Tax-Exempt Hospitals: Discussion Draft." Press release, Sen. Chuck Grassley, 2007. http://grassley.senate.gov/releases/2007/07182007.pdf (accessed Oct. 18, 2008).

Vigen, Aana Marie. *Women, Ethics, and Inequality in U.S. Healthcare: "To Count among the Living."* New York: Palgrave MacMillan, 2006.

Wallack, Stanley S., Cindy Parks Thomas, Signe Peterson Flieger, and Stuart H. Altman. "Massachusetts Health Care Cost Trends Part 1: The Massachusetts Health Care System in Context: Costs, Structure, and Methods Used by Private Insurers to Pay Providers," 2010. www.mass.gov/eohhs/docs/dhcfp/r/cost-trends-files/part1-system -in-context.pdf (accessed Oct. 29, 2012).

Walzer, Michael. *Spheres of Justice: A Defense of Pluralism and Equality*. New York: Basic Books, 1983.

Williams, David R. "Health and the Quality of Life of African Americans." In *The State of Black America*, edited by Lee A. Daniels, 115–38. New York: Urban League, 2004.

———. "The Health of U.S. Racial and Ethnic Populations." Special issue 2, *Journals of Gerontology* 60B (2005): 53–62.

Wilper, Andrew P., et al. "Health Insurance and Mortality in US Adults." *American Journal of Public Health* 99, no.12 (Dec. 2009): 2289–95.

Woolhandler, S., T. Campbell, and D. U. Himmelstein. "Health Care Administration Costs in the U.S. and Canada." *New England Journal of Medicine* 349 (Aug. 21, 2003): 768–75.

Woolhandler, Steffie, and David U. Himmelstein. "The New Massachusetts Health Reform: Half a Step Forward and Three Steps Back." *Hastings Center Report* 36, no. 5 (2006): 19–21.

Zoloth, Laurie. *Health Care and the Ethics of Encounter: A Jewish Discussion of Social Justice*. Chapel Hill: University of North Carolina, 1999.

Zoloth-Dorfman, Laurie. "An Ethics of Encounter: Public Choices and Private Acts." In Dorff and Newman, *Contemporary Jewish Ethics and Morality*, 219–45.

Court Cases and Legal Documents

Constitution of the State of Illinois. www.ilga.gov/commission/lrb/con9.htm (accessed Sept. 28, 2012).

Department of Health and Human Services, et al. v. Florida, et al. Oral Argument. United States Supreme Court Docket No. 11-398, Mar. 28, 2012. www.supremecourt.gov/oral_arguments/argument_transcripts/11-3 98-Tuesday.pdf (accessed June 5, 2012).

Internal Revenue Service. *IRS Exempt Organizations Hospital Compliance Project: Final Report.* www.irs.gov/pub/irs-tege/frepthospproj.pdf (accessed Sept. 27, 2012).

——. "Revenue Ruling 56-185," 1956. www.irs.gov/pub/irs-tege/rr56-185.pdf (accessed Oct. 18, 2008).

——. "Revenue Ruling 69-545," 1969. www.irs.gov/pub/irs-tege/rr69-545.pdf (accessed Oct. 18, 2008).

National Federation of Independent Businesses, et al. v. Sebelius, Secretary of Health and Human Services, et al. Supreme Court of the United States Docket No. 11-393, June 28, 2012. www.supremecourt.gov/opinions/11pdf/11-393c3a2.pdf (accessed June 28, 2012).

State of Florida v. United States Department of Health and Human Services. Case No. 3:10-cv-91-RV/EMT, Jan. 31, 2011. www.flnd.uscourts.gov/announcements/documents/10cv91doc150.pdf (accessed Feb. 10, 2012).

Tax-Exempt Hospital Responsibility Act. State of Illinois, HB5000 (2005 and 2006). www.ilga.gov/legislation/94/HB/PDF/09400HB5000lv.pdf (accessed Sept. 28, 2012).

Denominational Statements

Unless otherwise cited, all statements are from www.faithfulreform.org/ (accessed May 24, 2011).

Advisory Committee on Social Witness Policy, Presbyterian Church USA "Resolution on Advocacy on Behalf of the Uninsured," 2002. www.pcusa.org/resource/resolution-advocacy-behalf-uninsured/ (accessed June 30, 2011).

American Baptist Churches. "Health, Healing and Wholeness," 1991. www.abc-usa.org/wp-content/uploads/2012/06/health-healing-and-wholeness.pdf (accessed May 24, 2011).

——. "Resolution on Health Care for All," 1991.

Central Conference of American Rabbis. "National Health Care Resolution," 1991.

——. "Resolution on Health Care," 1976. http://rac.org/Articles/index.cfm?id=1825&pge_prg_id=15880&pge_id=2415 (accessed Aug. 18, 2012).

Church of the Brethren. "Health Care in the U.S.," 1989.

Church Women United. "Resolution on Universal Health Care," 1991.

Episcopal Church USA. "Health Care Coverage for All," 2009. In National Episcopal Health Ministries, *Healthy People, Healthy Church, Healthy Society*, appendix 6.

————. "Right of All Individuals to Comprehensive Health Care," 1991.

Evangelical Lutheran Church in America. "Caring for Health: Our Shared Endeavor," 2003. www.elca.org/what-we-believe/social-issues/social-statements/health-and-health care.aspx (accessed June 29, 2011).

Leadership Council of Conservative Judaism. "National Health Care," 1992. http://uscj2004.aptinet.com/Judaism_and_health_C5336.html (accessed July 7, 2011).

————. "For the Health of the Nation: An Evangelical Call to Civic Responsibility," 2004. www.nae.net/images/content/for_the_health _of_the_nation.pdf (accessed July 1, 2011).

National Association of Evangelicals. "Health Care Reform," 1994; reaffirmed in 2009. www.nae.net/government-relations/policy-resolutions/174-health-care-reform-1994 (accessed July 5, 2011).

National Council of Churches of Christ. "Renewed Faith Community Universal Health Care Campaign," 1999.

National Episcopal Health Ministries. *Healthy People, Healthy Church, Healthy Society*, 2006. www.episcopalhealthministries.org/resources/health-care (accessed July 5, 2011).

National Federation of Temple Sisterhoods. "Universal Access to Health Care," 1991.

Religious Action Center of Reform Judaism. "Reform Judaism and Universal Health Care" (2002).

Southern Baptist Convention. "Resolution on Health Care Reform," June 1994. www .sbc.net/resolutions/amResolution.asp?ID = 594 (accessed July 5, 2011).

Standing Commission on Health, Episcopal Church USA. "Christians and the Formation of Public Policy about Health Care." In National Episcopal Health Ministries, *Healthy People, Healthy Church, Healthy Society*, 25–30.

United Church of Christ. "An Urgent Call for Advocacy in Support for Health Care for All," 2009. www.ucc.org/justice/health/pdfs/corrected-resolution-on-Single-payer -Jan-09.pdf (accessed June 30, 2011).

United Methodist Church. "Universal Health Care in the United States of America," 2001.

US Conference of Catholic Bishops. "A Framework for Comprehensive Reform: Protecting Human Life, Promoting Human Dignity, Pursuing the Common Good," 1993. http://old.usccb.org/sdwp/national/comphealth.shtml (accessed Nov. 20, 2010).

Index

abortion and the ACA, 5, 60, 61, 68–69

ACA. *See* Affordable Care Act (ACA)

access to health care, 12–13, 47–48, 50

accountability. *See* community accountability

accountable care organizations (ACOs), 150, 224

Affordable Care Act (ACA), 17–18, 214–37; abortion funding, 5, 60, 61, 68–69; balancing charity and justice, 229–32; balancing mercy and truth, 228–29; birth control mandate, 5, 21n8, 22n11; and broader social responsibility in health care, 147–48; building on existing social structures, 209–10; and community accountability, 104; and community benefits/uncompensated care debate, 146–51, 230–31; cost-control measures, 65, 214, 220–21, 224; critics' analogies to challenge constitutionality, 52n25; dignity and stewardship, 232–36; and DSH payments, 104; employer mandate, 219–20, 236n10; and FQHCs, 100, 102, 104; free preventive services, 221; health care reform debate, 1–2, 17–18, 27, 179, 183–84; implementation, 1, 183; individual mandate, 12, 50, 63, 113–17, 148, 208–10, 219–20, 236n10; and market reformers' emphasis on individual preferences, 216–19; and Medicaid, 45, 48, 104, 110, 119, 119n43, 149, 186, 219, 221; and Medicare Advantage plans, 221; and Medicare IPAB, 216, 217, 221–22; objections based on view of health care as private benefit, 31–32, 224; and Oregon's Medicaid reforms, 10, 215–16, 225; overview of policy tools and goals, 20, 214–37; PCORI, 222; popular opinion, 212n1; and POSHs, 173, 221; provision against insurance denials for preexisting conditions, 50, 209; and public-private partnership model, 222–25; religious objections, 5, 21n8, 60, 61, 68–69; required statements of employer-paid premiums and health savings contributions, 51n10; and social responsiveness, 147–49; and social stewardship, 20, 219–25; solidarity and moral imperative, 179, 185; subsidies for low-to moderate-income Americans, 12, 40, 209; Supreme Court oral arguments, 114–16; Supreme Court ruling, 1, 27, 208–10; and Tea Party movement, 183–84

Affordable Care Today! (ACT) coalition, 184

African Americans: breast cancer screening protocols and hospital transparency, 174–75; health disparities, 63–64

Akiva, Rabbi, 71

Altman, Stuart, 222

American Baptist Churches, 56, 73, 74

American Enterprise Institute, 188

American exceptionalism, emphasis on personal liberty, 17, 31, 78, 183-84, 200-201, 216

American Medical Association (AMA), 105–6, 118n25

American Recovery and Reinvestment Act, 102

Arrow, Kenneth J., 22n21

255